Dedication...

To all those who have struggled with "not feeling right", knowing that your hormones are out of balance… and have fought the good battles but feel like you are losing the war, I dedicate this book to you.

It's not your fault and you are not alone.

I am grateful to God for what I call, "allowing things to happen **for** me and not **to** me", as these personal experiences and trials with my own hormone imbalance issues have led me to be able to help you.

To all those patients who have taught me, through precious trial and process, what to do and what not to do, I thank you that others can learn from your journey. To my son, **Donnie**, my "Why".

Dr. Tammy Tucker
213 West Monroe Suite P Lowell AR 72745

Second Edition

Printed in the USA
Lily Grace Publishing, INC
ISBN-13: 978-1502967879

ISBN-10: 1502967871

Table of Contents

Introduction

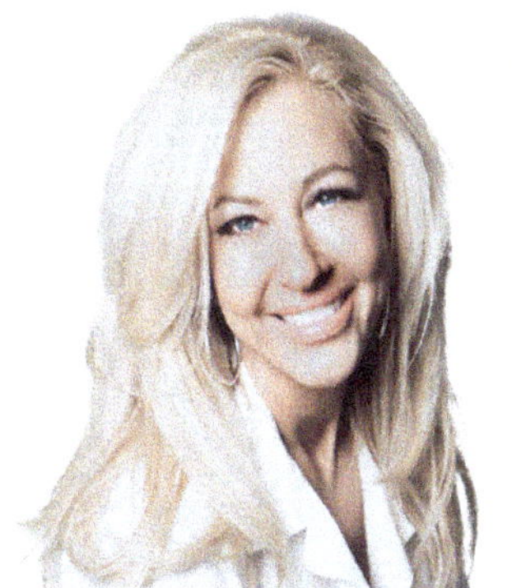

Welcome to your go-to guide on the often misunderstood conductors of your life's internal orchestra - **Hormones.**

I'm Dr. Tammy, the "Hormone Queen," and I've dedicated over 24 years to unmasking the secrets behind living your healthiest life!

Here are some of the things we're going to take a deep dive into...

Hormones: The Unsung Heroes (or Villains)

Think of hormones as the string section in your body's grand symphony. When all is well, you feel like you're floating on cloud nine, but let one violin—er, hormone—get out of tune, and you can feel like you're living in a never-ending Monday.

How Do You Know It's Your Hormones?

Are you familiar with that nagging thought, "Could my hormones be out of whack?" Or have you been ever-so-gently nudged by someone who cares, asking, "Have you thought about getting your hormones checked, honey?" You're not alone. This book is for everyone who's asked that question, for those who've been told "You're fine," or even worse, "It's not your hormones." Maddening, right?

Intuition Meets Science

If you're questioning if it's your hormones, it most likely is. After all, these biochemical wizards govern everything from how much weight you gain to those mysterious mood swings. But hey, it's not your fault. You're in good company, and this book is your first step towards regaining your balance and vitality.

Your Personal Roadmap

Want the best starting point for balancing those pesky hormones? I usually have my patients complete a comprehensive questionnaire. This invaluable tool helps me see you—not just as a chart or a number—but as a beautifully complex individual. We'll combine that insight with lab tests to tailor-make your hormone harmonizing plan.

Continued...

This is more than just another health book.

it's your guide to liberation.

We're diving into regenerative and integrative medicine, breaking down complex hormonal hieroglyphics into digestible wisdom.

Imagine a life where you wake up energized, your weight is just a number, and mood swings are a thing of the past. Sound heavenly?

It's entirely possible, and your map to that life is in these pages.

So buckle up, buttercup! Grab your favorite herbal tea, get cozy, and let's navigate the sometimes bewildering but always fascinating world of hormones together.

We're not just cracking the code; we're reclaiming your life--one hormone at a time.

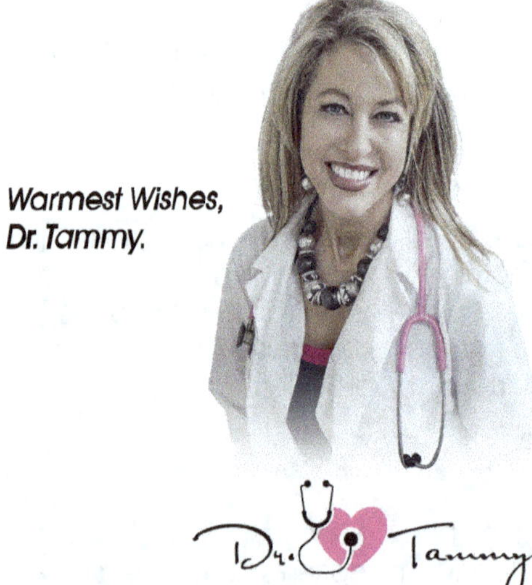

Warmest Wishes,
Dr. Tammy.

Oh! There's one other thing...

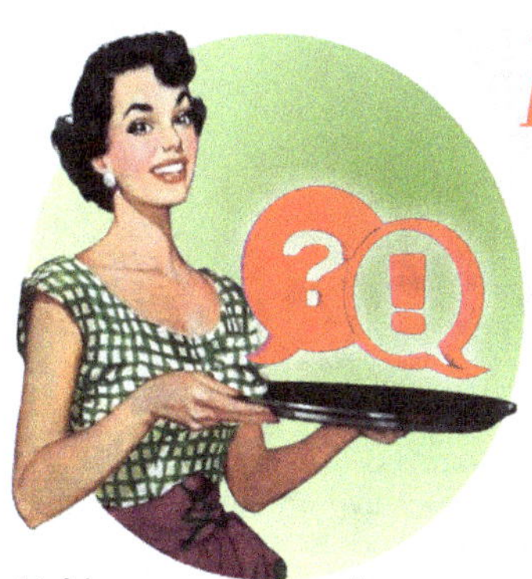

Hormone Myths

Dispelling the Fears and Fiction

"Let's just get this out of the way!"

Hold on to your seats, because we're about to turn some long-standing myths upside down! We're going to clear the cobwebs and set the record straight on hormones, one myth at a time.

As we dig deep, you'll discover not just the what, but also the why behind these misconceptions.Now, if you've been on this hormone-balancing journey with me for a while, you might think you're immune to the old myths.

But guess what?

Even seasoned pros can get rattled. Let's face it, well-meaning family and friends can sometimes knock us off our well-researched pedestals with outdated information.

Who hasn't received a frantic call or text warning us that our bio-identical hormones are going to give us this or that dreadful disease?

Yes, I still get those calls from my patients. Even if they've experienced transformative health benefits from their hormone therapy, the moment someone whispers the words **"breast cancer"** or **"heart disease,"** panic sets in.

I get it.

These myths have been around for a long time, and **fear** is a **powerful** thing.

So let's tackle this head-on.

I've compiled a list of the *10 most persistent, pesky myths* that just keep making the rounds.

This list is your go-to guide when doubt starts to creep in, or when you need to set the record straight with a well-intentioned friend.

Let's jump in and bust these myths wide open, shall we?

Because knowledge is power, and you deserve to make health decisions based on **facts, not fear.**

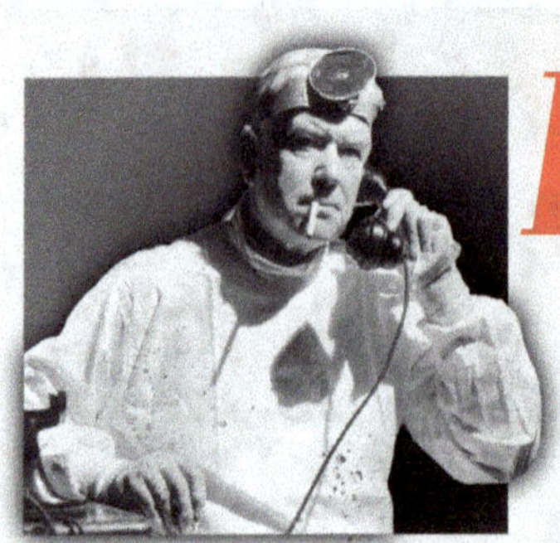

Ten Hormone Myths

keep this list on hand or even stick it on your fridge! It's your go-to guide for setting the record straight when those hormone myths start rearing their ugly heads

All Hormones Cause Cancer: A fear-mongering classic! Actually, bio-identical hormones have different physiological effects than synthetic ones.

Testosterone is Just for Men: No way, Jose! Women also need testosterone for muscle mass, bone density, and even mental clarity.

Estrogen is Bad for You: A one-sided tale. There are different types of estrogen, and imbalance is what causes problems, not estrogen itself.

Hormone Therapy is Only for Post-Menopausal Women: Nope, hormone imbalances can happen at any age and affect both genders. Early intervention is key!

Bioidentical Hormones are a Marketing Gimmick: Oh, please! These hormones are structurally identical to the ones your body makes, which often makes them more effective and better tolerated.

Progesterone and Progestin are the Same: Don't mix these up! Progestin is synthetic and does not have the full range of benefits that natural progesterone offers.

Thyroid Issues are Easy to Diagnose with a TSH Test: If only it were that simple! Comprehensive tests that look at T3, T4, and reverse T3 are also crucial for an accurate diagnosis.

Adrenal Fatigue is a Made-Up Condition: Tell that to someone who's constantly stressed and tired! While it might not be recognized universally, HPA axis dysregulation is a real issue.

If You're on Hormones, You Don't Need Lifestyle Changes: Yeah, right! Hormone therapy works best in conjunction with a balanced diet, regular exercise, and stress management.

You Can Self-Medicate with Over-the-Counter Hormone Creams: Tread carefully! Hormones are potent messengers and you need the right tests and professional guidance for effective, safe treatment.

Before we dive deeper into the maze of hormones, let's arm ourselves with a trusty map...

...disguised as a questionnaire.

Chapter 1

You might be wondering, "Why do I need to fill out a checklist? Can't I just read along and get the info I need?"

HORMONE IMBALANCE SYMPTOMS CHECKLIST

This questionnaire serves multiple purposes:

Self-Awareness: It helps you take stock of your symptoms and how they fluctuate, painting a more comprehensive picture of your hormonal landscape.

Guidepost: Think of it as mile markers on a highway. These symptoms will guide you to relevant sections in the book, making your journey more focused and less overwhelming.

Progress Tracker: As you implement changes, you can revisit the questionnaire to gauge your progress. Nothing is more satisfying than ticking off symptoms you no longer experience!

MILD, MOD, SEVERE

PMS (premenstrual syndrome) issues, such as cramps, nausea, breast tenderness, headaches, and/or irritability 2-1 weeks before my period.

MILD, MOD, SEVERE

Difficulty falling asleep or staying asleep

MILD, MOD, SEVERE

Fatigue or loss of energy especially in the afternoon.

MILD, MOD, SEVERE

Frequent bouts of irritability and depression.

MILD, MOD, SEVERE

Frequent anxious feelings, anxiety attacks, or heart palpitations

MILD, MOD, SEVERE

Achy or stiff joints, especially in the morning

MILD, MOD, SEVERE

Gaining weight. especially around the middle

MILD, MOD, SEVERE

Difficulty losing weight

MILD, MOD, SEVERE

Pain with intercourse

MILD, MOD, SEVERE

Inability to have orgasm, decreased sensitivity, or sex drive

MILD, MOD, SEVERE

Vaginal dryness

MILD, MOD, SEVERE

Crave sweets, carbohydrates or alcohol

MILD, MOD, SEVERE

Dry, fragile, or thinning skin and hair

MILD, MOD, SEVERE

Losing height. diagnosed w/osteoporosis, broken or fractured bones

MILD, MOD, SEVERE

Irregular menstrual periods

MILD, MOD, SEVERE

Hot flashes or night sweats

MILD, MOD, SEVERE

Missing the outer third of your eyebrows

HORMONE IMBALANCE SYMPTOMS CHECKLIST

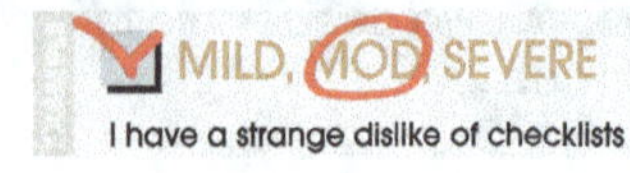

MILD, MOD, SEVERE
Frequent headaches or migraines

MILD, MOD, SEVERE
Fluid retention (rings fit tight or shoe size increased)

MILD, MOD, SEVERE
History of cysts on ovaries

MILD, MOD, SEVERE
Facial hair, male pattern balding

MILD, MOD, SEVERE
Intolerance to heat or cold

MILD, MOD, SEVERE
Excessive sweating

MILD, MOD, SEVERE
Changes in voice or hoarseness

MILD, MOD, SEVERE
Reduced sense of taste or smell

MILD, MOD, SEVERE
Rapid heartbeat or palpitations

MILD, MOD, SEVERE
Acne or oily skin

MILD, MOD, SEVERE
Dark circles under the eyes

MILD, MOD, SEVERE
Changes in appetite

MILD, MOD, SEVERE
Problems with acne or rosacea

MILD, MOD, SEVERE
Heart racing or irregular heartbeats felt

MILD, MOD, SEVERE
Hot or cold intolerance

MILD, MOD, SEVERE
Constipation or diarrhea

MILD, MOD, SEVERE
Frequent bouts of abdominal bloating or gas

MILD, MOD, SEVERE
Skin rash or new onset allergies

MILD, MOD, SEVERE
Brittle Nails

MILD, MOD, SEVERE
Brain fog

MILD, MOD, SEVERE
Feeling cold often

MILD, MOD, SEVERE
Excessive thirst and urination

MILD, MOD, SEVERE
Excessive urination

MILD, MOD, SEVERE
Sensitivity to light or sound

MILD, MOD, SEVERE
Mood swings

HOW DO YOU FEEL?

HORMONE IMBALANCE SYMPTOMS CHECKLIST

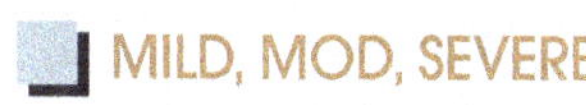

MILD, MOD, SEVERE
Lightheadedness or dizziness

MILD, MOD, SEVERE
High blood pressure

MILD, MOD, SEVERE
Frequent colds or infections

MILD, MOD, SEVERE
Persistent digestive issues

MILD, MOD, SEVERE
Intolerance to heat or cold

MILD, MOD, SEVERE
Nausea or lack of appetite

MILD, MOD, SEVERE
Tingling or numbness in extremities

MILD, MOD, SEVERE
Excessive or reduced body hair

MILD, MOD, SEVERE
Dry eyes

MILD, MOD, SEVERE
Recurring skin rashes or eczema

MILD, MOD, SEVERE
Cold hands and feet

MILD, MOD, SEVERE
Frequent blushing or flushing

MILD, MOD, SEVERE
Bruising easily

MILD, MOD, SEVERE
Sleep apnea or snoring

MILD, MOD, SEVERE
Shortness of breath

MILD, MOD, SEVERE
Loss of libido

MILD, MOD, SEVERE
Sudden or unexplained weight loss

MILD, MOD, SEVERE
Tinnitus (ringing in the ears)

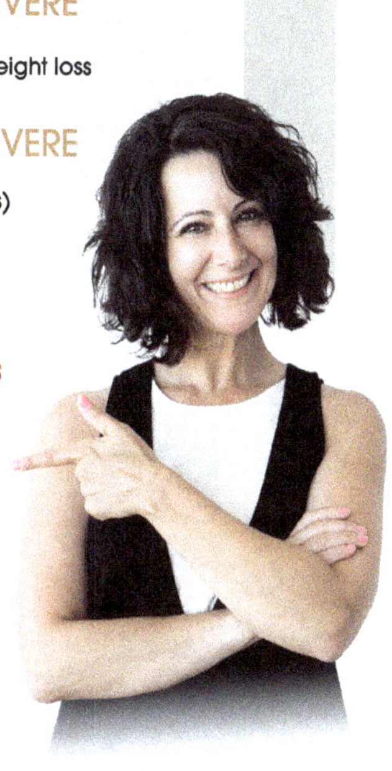

Remember, it's essential to be as accurate as possible when filling this out.

Your answers will not only help you understand your unique needs but will also make your trip through this book more fruitful.

With this personalized roadmap, we're well on our way to achieving the balance you've been longing for!

Notes...

CHAPTER 2

My Awakening: A Doctor's Personal Journey Into The World of Hormones

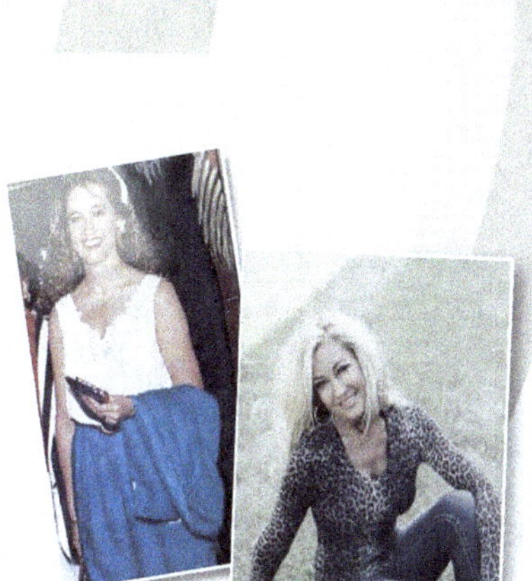

Imagine my astonishment when, after 13 years of trying, I unexpectedly found myself pregnant! I carried my baby to term, but the journey was fraught with severe complications that had me teetering on the edge in the ICU. Those steroid medications, necessary for my survival, had me gain over seventy pounds—I was unrecognizable to myself. And even months postpartum, I was still squeezing into my maternity clothes.

Breastfeeding helped me shed some weight, but it felt like a drop in an ocean of health issues. The weight of never-ending hunger was almost too much to bear, not to mention the resumption of heavier-than-ever periods. A nagging pain on my right side finally drove me to seek an ultrasound. The results? Multiple fibroid tumors and a suspicious mass on my right ovary. The alarm bells of potential cancer rang loud in my ears, and so, feeling cornered, I chose a hysterectomy.

I thought I'd find relief, but life threw another curveball: hot flashes! My adrenal glands acted up; my thyroid gave up on me; my weight skyrocketed again.

Yes, you heard that right.

A doctor with no clue about her own body's intricate dance of hormones.

Sure, biology and physiology classes taught me the 'what,' but they never touched upon the 'how' - the profound impact of hormones on our well-being.

Enter a game-changing patient, sophisticated and articulate, who casually dropped the question, "Do you prescribe bioidentical hormones?"

"Bio-what?" I blinked.

The conversation that followed was nothing short of an epiphany. This patient shattered all my preconceived notions—nay, misconceptions—about hormone replacement therapy (HRT). Her enlightening words set me on a path to self-discovery and catalyzed an urgent need to expand my horizons as a physician.

Some doctors, overwhelmed with the rigors of modern medicine, ask, "Why venture outside the familiar lanes of big pharma?"

I have a simple answer: Because my patients deserve better.

The Google search bar became my portal to a new world - a world of bioidentical hormones.

Fast forward eight years: I've lost sixty pounds, said goodbye to night sweats and hot flashes, and rediscovered my zest for life.

My newfound understanding also gave me a deeper perspective on how unnecessary my hysterectomy likely was. My fibroids, my endometriosis, and even my heavy periods were all messengers of a deeper issue: Hormonal imbalance.
I've been fortunate to witness transformations that are nothing short of miracles: pounds melting away, relationships rejuvenating, lives reclaiming their sparkle—all thanks to hormonal balance. So, I dedicate myself to this path, armed with a commitment to keep digging deeper, because you deserve a healthcare partner who will go the

I've been fortunate to witness transformations that are nothing short of miracles:

pounds melting away

relationships rejuvenating

lives reclaiming their sparkle

all thanks to hormonal balance.

So, I dedicate myself to this path, armed with a commitment to keep digging deeper, because you deserve a healthcare partner who will go the extra mile.

The principles behind achieving hormonal harmony are fundamentally simple, albeit the nuances are complex.

That's what this book is about: ***decoding the complex so that you can live your life—not just exist, but truly LIVE.***

Until that point, I ***believed*** a woman didn't need progesterone if she didn't have a uterus. I was taught there was only one way to take hormone replacement therapy and only a couple of different options or doses.

I told my patient I knew nothing about what she was talking about, and I promised her I would find out.

I try to keep an open mind about alternative therapies   although many physicians don't because there is already so much to learn and know.

Why add more?

These physicians ask, "If there is no evidence-based research behind it (or at least that's what big pharmaceutical companies would have us believe), isn't it better to prescribe a pill?" Some doctors cattle forty or more patients through their halls a day. That doesn't leave much time to look into alternative therapies.

I feel very differently about this and for this reason I vowed to look into "bioidentical hormone therapy".

I googled Suzanne and soon had unlocked a door to a world I never knew existed That was eight years ago. So, what was the outcome?

I started on bioidentical hormone therapy (and I prescribed it for that patient, too).

I lost over sixty pounds and escaped night sweats and hot flashes! My mood was stable for once and I was sleeping again.

I put testosterone in the prescription and actually got a libido back that might have saved my marriage. I felt better than I had felt since those nasty periods started when I was a teenager.

I learned that my hysterectomy was probably not necessary. The abnormal pap, fibroids, and endometriosis found at the time of my surgery were all a product of my massive hormone imbalances.

I learned my heavy periods were from the excess estrogen I was storing, when I unknowingly put on an extra 10 lbs in college.

From this and more, I have learned patients do not have to suffer and have unnecessary procedures, surgeries and rely on big pharmaceutical companies' answers to these issues.

Over the past eight years, I have seen patients lose hundreds of pounds. People have transformed before my very eyes. Marriages have been healed from the ravages of hormonally imbalanced women AND men. I have been given a gift to be able to help people through this journey. I have sought out every aspect of metabolic realignment I could and this is the simplest presentation I have come up with. The principles are really quite simple, although the nuances can be tricky. You will need a physician on your side willing to go the distance and pay attention to the details.

gift to be able to help people through this journey. I have sought out every aspect of metabolic realignment I could and this is the simplest presentation I have come up with.

The principles are really quite simple, although the nuances can be tricky.

You will need a physician on your side willing to go the distance and pay attention to the details.

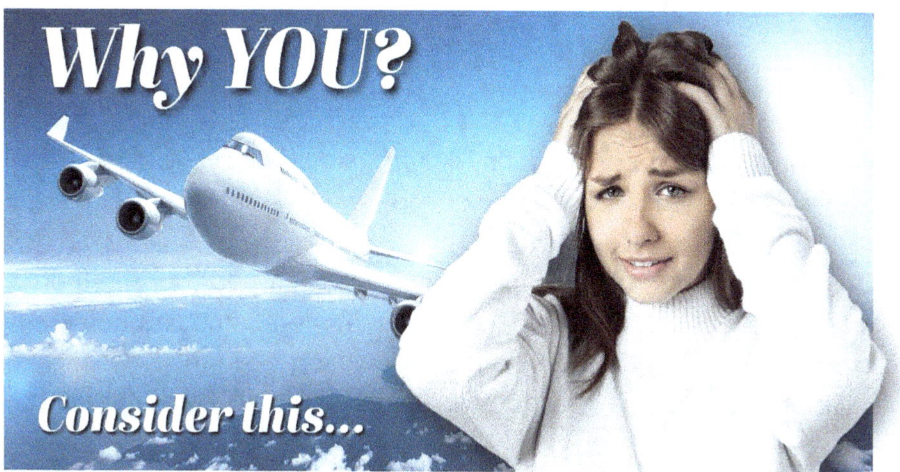

Imagine you're on an airplane, cruising at 30,000 feet, and **suddenly the cabin pressure drops.**

The oxygen masks drop down from above your seat.

The first thing you're instructed to do is to put on your own mask before assisting others.

Why?

Because if you're gasping for air, you're in no condition to help anyone else.

The same holds true for hormonal balance and overall health. If your hormones are out of whack, you're essentially operating at a low "cabin pressure." You might feel fatigued, stressed, or emotionally volatile; it's like trying to breathe in a cabin with low oxygen. Your ability

If your hormones are out of whack, you're essentially operating at a low "cabin pressure." You might feel fatigued, stressed, or emotionally volatile...

...it's like trying to breathe in a cabin with low oxygen.

Your ability to care for your family, excel in your career, or even simply enjoy life's pleasures is severely compromised.

Putting yourself first isn't selfish;.

It's foundational.

Balancing your hormones is akin to putting on that oxygen mask. It allows you to breathe easier, think clearer, and live better.

Only then are you truly equipped to help those around you. Whether it's playing with your kids without feeling drained, being emotionally present with your partner, or nailing that work presentation, having balanced hormones is your ticket to succeeding in all areas of your life.

So, secure your "oxygen mask" **first** by getting your hormones checked and balanced.

It's not just a favor to yourself; **it's a gift to everyone who relies on you.**

Notes...

CHAPTER 3

How Did I Get Like This?!

Well, let's start by saying that *it's not your fault.* You may have made some decisions that lead to these issues but probably made those decisions unaware of what you were doing to your body.

This is an appropriate answer for the question that many patients ask: "How did I get like this?" Dayafter day the average American participates in an all-out onslaught on their own health. Overwork, physical and mental overstrain, sleep deprivation, noise pollution, late hours, surgery, medications, injuries, inflammation, pain, toxicity, ingestion of chemicals, poor diet filled with packaged and processed non-nutritive foods, electromagnetic fields, poor digestion, blood sugar issues, environmental *xenohormones*, allergies, and the list goes on and on.

We did not even talk about emotional stressors.

Oh, we just did.

All of these insults to our systems lead to endocrine disruption and hormone imbalances. When we chronically don't take proper care of our
systems, they begin to malfunction. Your body may require more of
one hormone in a certain instance. When that hormone increases over
a period of time, others will begin to decrease leading to   imbalance. Allow this strain of the system to go on long enough and you
have a full scale war going on inside of you, and you are the   benefac-

Female hormone imbalance is rampant in our country.

It affects nearly all women at one time or another in their lives.

Indirectly, it affects us all! It is reported that 60% of American women suffer from PMS.

Ah, PMS! It's like that unwelcome party guest that shows up every
month, isn't it? Medically speaking, PMS stands for Premenstrual
Syndrome. It's a collection of symptoms that many women experience
about 1 to 2 weeks before their menstrual period starts.

Imagine your hormones playing musical chairs in your body; things can
get a bit chaotic!

So, what's in the PMS grab bag? Oh, a delightful mix of emotional,
psychological, and physical symptoms. You might experience mood
swings, irritability, or even depression. It's like riding an emotional rollercoaster without having bought a ticket for it. Physically, you could be
grappling with bloating, breast tenderness, and headaches. Yep, the
works!

Why does it happen, you ask? Well, it's a bit like your body throwing a
mini-revolt as it prepares for menstruation.

Your hormone levels fluctuate, particularly estrogen and progesterone,
and this upheaval is what triggers those delightful symptoms. Picture
your hormone levels like a see-saw - when they're not balanced
everything feels a bit wobbly.

Thankfully, PMS is usually predictable (it has a schedule, sort of like a recurring villain in a superhero series). So, with a bit of smart lifestyle management (**think exercise, balanced nutrition, and stress control**) you can often manage or reduce the symptoms.

Everything is about BALANCE! I guess you are starting to see that...

Oh, let's dive right into estrogen dominance, shall we?

Before we do, we need to define what the word ovulate means:

Ovulation is like the VIP event in a woman's menstrual cycle. Imagine your ovaries rolling out the red carpet once a month for a special egg.

During this time, usually around the middle of your menstrual cycle, one of your ovaries releases a mature egg that travels down the fallopian tube, making its grand entrance and waiting for a sperm to fertilize it.

If it doesn't meet its "Mr. Right" sperm within about 12 to 24 hours, the egg dissolves, and then you start the whole cycle again with your next period.

In short, ovulation is when an egg is released from the ovary and it's the time when you're most fertile. If you're tracking your menstrual cycle for pregnancy or contraceptive reasons, this is a critical time to know about.

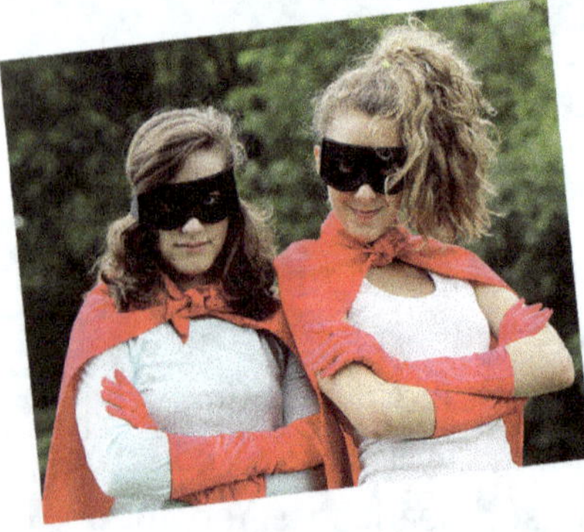

Think of estrogen and progesterone like a dynamic duo working to keep everything in your body running smoothly.

But what happens when Batman suddenly has way too many gadgets and Robin can't keep up? Chaos!

That's what estrogen dominance is like - it's when estrogen starts hogging the limelight, either because its levels have skyrocketed or because progesterone has dipped low.

Imagine it like missing a key player in a sports game - when you don't ovulate, no progesterone gets produced. It's like trying to bake a cake but forgetting the sugar; things just don't turn out right.

This sets the stage for estrogen to take the lead, and not in a good way.

So, why might a woman not ovulate?

One big culprit is stress.

Think of your adrenal glands like your body's battery. Chronic stress can drain this battery, leading to all sorts of hormonal mayhem, like estrogen dominance. This can result in things like wonky menstrual cycles, periods that are too long or too short, and yep, you guessed it - no ovulation.

Now, how do you know if you're dealing with estrogen dominance? While proper testing is the gold standard (like going to a mechanic for an expert diagnosis), symptoms might include mood swings, weight gain, and headaches.

In simpler terms, if you feel like you're on a never-ending hormonal rollercoaster, it might be worth getting checked out.

Calculating it is usually a matter of ratios - comparing the levels of estrogen and progesterone in your body. It's like measuring the ingredients for a cocktail; you want the perfect balance to make it taste just right. *But, I gotta emphasize, this isn't a DIY project - consult a healthcare provider to get accurate lab interpretations.*

Just for a little understanding if you want a little nerdy science here, lets jump in to it:

The essence of the information is that balancing estrogen and progesterone is like a delicate dance - both partners have to be in sync. When they're not, you start experiencing symptoms, even if each hormone level appears "normal" on its own. Let's break it down into bite-sized pieces:

Imagine estrogen and progesterone are like two dancers on a stage. When one takes the spotlight too much, the performance feels off. This spotlight-stealing is what we call an "imbalance."

I once had a patient present with hot flashes and was newly postmenopausal. Her first test showed a low ratio, so we started her on topical progesterone.

It worked wonders!

Fast forward, and her symptoms returned. **Why?** Her ratio got too high because her estrogen levels had dropped. She could either reduce her progesterone, increase estrogen, or adjust both to get back to feeling fabulous.

So there you go! Understanding your hormone ratio is like knowing the secret handshake in the club of hormonal balance. It helps you and your healthcare provider decide the next steps in your treatment, whether you're just starting on your hormone journey or you're a seasoned traveler.

Estrogen dominance is like that friend at a party who doesn't know when to call it quits - fun in moderation but overwhelming when there's too much.

Just like you wouldn't want one friend to hog all the limelight, you wouldn't want estrogen to overshadow its partner, progesterone.

When estrogen hogs the hormonal stage, it can lead to a range of symptoms like bloating, irregular menstrual cycles, fatigue, and even mood swings. In the long run, estrogen dominance can open the door to more serious issues like fibroids, endometriosis, and even certain cancers.

Knowing if you're tipping the scales towards estrogen dominance is crucial. It's like having a weather forecast for your body - you'll know when to carry an umbrella to shield yourself from a hormonal downpour.

Even small lifestyle changes in diet, stress management, and exercise can help restore the balance, but first, you've gotta know what you're up against.

MOOD SWINGS

Awareness is the first step towards reclaiming your hormonal harmony!

- [ ] Yup, more rollercoasters than an amusement park!
- [ ] Nope, I'm as stable as they come.

IRREGULAR PERIODS

- [ ] My cycle has a mind of its own.
- [ ] Like clockwork, every month.

CHRONIC FATIGUE

- [ ] I could sleep for days...
- [ ] Energized and ready to go!

WEIGHT GAIN

- [ ] My jeans are feeling the pinch!
- [ ] Weight's staying consistent.

BLOATING & WATER RETENTION

- [ ] I feel like a human water balloon!
- [ ] No puffiness here.

FIBROCYSTIC BREASTS

- [ ] Lumps and discomfort.
- [ ] All's normal in that department

LOW LIBIDO

- [ ] Where did my mojo go?
- [ ] Still got that spark

If you've checked more than three of the scary choices, it might be time to consult a healthcare provider and consider getting your hormone levels tested.

"Now, I know some of you are thinking, 'Hold on, Dr. Tammy, I've already crossed the peri-menopause finish line, and I'm chilling in the 'no-more-periods' VIP lounge!' Well, cheers to you!

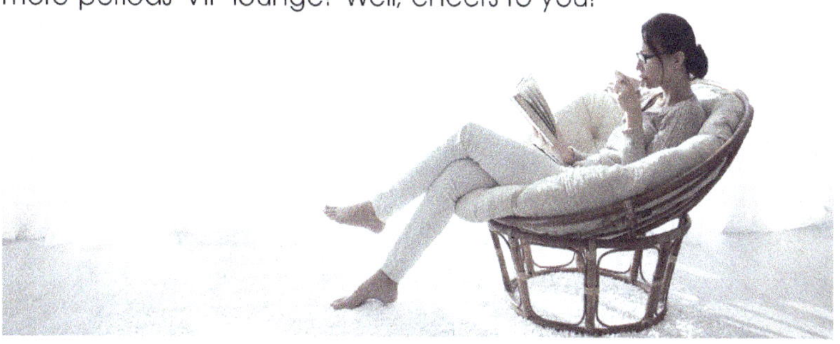

But don't tune out just yet. Whether you're a teenager just stepping into the hormonal rollercoaster, in the thick of peri-menopause, or you've already thrown your periods a retirement party, all of this information is still golden. Trust me, your hormones are like the cast of a long-running TV show—they go through different seasons, sure, but the storyline is interconnected. So whether you're in Season 1 or Season 7 of your hormonal journey, this is must-see TV!"

I know some of you might be thinking, "Well, I'm not having periods anymore, so why should I care about all this?"

Trust me, whether you're in your early menstruation years, navigating the unpredictable seas of peri-menopause, or have sailed into the territory of menopause, this information is like your North Star. It's guiding you through the often murky waters of hormonal changes.

So hang tight! By the end of this book, you'll become the *Hormone Whisperer* - armed with the knowledge to not only understand your body better but also to assist those around you.

Your daughters, granddaughters, sisters, and friends are all riding this hormonal roller coaster at different speeds, **and the more you know, the more you become the superhero of your tribe.**

Imagine being the go-to guru who knows why Aunt Jane is always hot-flashing or why your best friend can't sleep. You could be the difference between years of struggling and a faster path to feeling fabulous!

So let's continue, shall we?

Together, we're going to unravel the mysteries, debunk the myths, and get you well on your way to **hormonal harmony.**

Progesterone's job is two-fold: 1) to prepare the uterus for implantation with a healthy fertilized egg, and 2) to support the early stage of pregnancy. If no implantation occurs, progesterone levels drop until another cycle begins.

Studies have shown that progesterone has anti-proliferative effects on breast cancer and leukemia cells. Breast cancer is 5,4 times more common in pre menopausal women with low progesterone levels than with favorable levels (Cowan 1981).

Data suggest that while bioidentical (i.e., natural) progesterone does not increase risk of breast cancer, synthetic progestins used in conventional HRT do.

Natural progesterone has also demonstrated neuro-protective properties. One study called for more attention to progesterone as a "potent neurotrophic agent that may play an important role in reducing or preventing motor, cognitive, and sensory impairments (in both men and women)".

THE DIFFERENCE IN CHEMICAL STRUCTURE IS OBVIOUS...

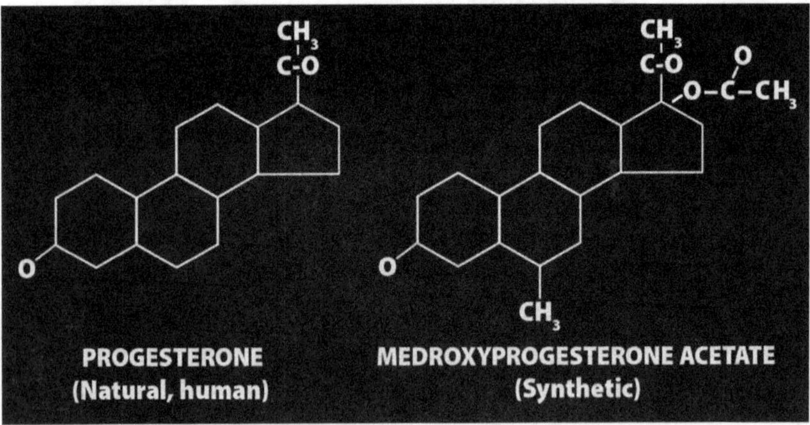

The difference in structure can promote a pregnancy (pro-gestation) and keep a woman who has had difficulty carrying a pregnancy to term, versus synthetic which can cause a miscarriage (DEATH) to a fetus!

Notes...

Chapter 4

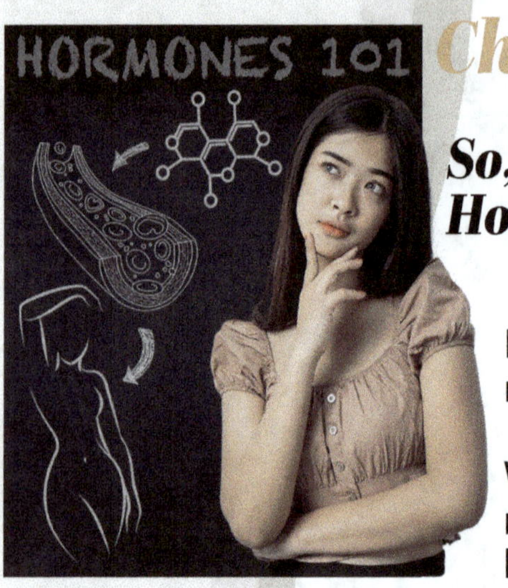

So, What Are Hormones?

Let's kick it off with a "Hormones 101" course, shall we?

We're going to unravel the mysteries surrounding these biochemical superstars and unravel the mystery of hormones and demystify them as well as *debunk* the *myths* like:

ESTROGEN IS BAD
and
ALL HORMONES ARE ESTROGEN.

> ***The term "hormone" actually hails from the Greek word 'horman,' meaning "to urge on" or "impulse." It's like the cheerleader for your body, rooting for specific actions or changes.***

We All Need Hormones. Just as we need oxygen to live (yes, we're all "addicted" to it), hormones are another non-negotiable for life. I've had emphysema patients hesitant to use supplemental oxygen because they're afraid of getting addicted. Let's clear the air: we're all oxygen addicts by necessity!

Hormones are like the strings of a finely-tuned guitar; each has a role, and balance is key. One isn't more critical than the other; they work in harmony. Just as a guitar has different chords, our hormones have their highs and lows throughout the day, following our circadian rhythms.

You're basically a walking, talking, shopping symphony of hormones! These fantastic little messengers regulate everything from how you feel to what you do. It's like having an internal software system that dictates all your operations.

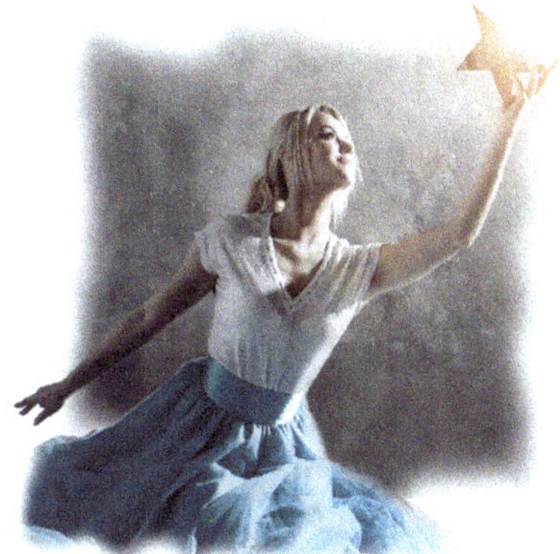

The Stars of the Show

For example, **estrogen** is the diva that makes us 'girly,' helping females go through puberty, maintaining menstrual cycles, and even contributing to libido and breast health.

By understanding hormones, we not only get insights into our bodily functions but also open doors to better health and wellness.

So let's dive deeper and look at the roles of various hormones and the effects they have on us.

Picture hormones as the text messages of the body. They're little chemical messengers that zip around, telling your cells what to do, when to do it, and how much of it needs to be done. Like getting an emoji-filled text from a friend that says, "Party at my place!" Your cells jump into action, just like you would, pulling on your party shoes.

Now, where do these hormones come from? Think of hormone-producing glands like tiny, specialized factories in your body.

Some of the big players are the pituitary gland, the thyroid, and the adrenal glands, among others. Each factory specializes in making certain types of hormones, and they're really good at it!

Imagine a "mood factory" churning out serotonin and dopamine, while another "growth factory" is busy making hormones that help you grow tall or build muscles.

The creation of hormones is a fascinating blend of science and magic - well, biochemistry, to be exact!

Let's say the brain senses that you need more energy because you're running a marathon. It sends a signal to the adrenal glands, like hitting the "emergency" button, and voila! They produce adrenaline, your body's very own "turbo-charge," giving you that extra oomph to cross the finish line.

Once these hormones are made, they take a trip through the bloodstream—imagine them catching the Hormone Express. They travel until they find the specific cells they're designed to chat with, also known as target cells. When they arrive, they bind to these cells like a key fitting into a lock, triggering them into action. It's like showing an exclusive VIP pass at a concert; they get access to initiate all kinds of fun and essential activities in the body.

By understanding hormones, we not only get insights into our bodily functions but also open doors to better health and wellness.

So let's dive deeper and look at the roles of various hormones and the effects they have on us.

Picture hormones as the text messages of the body. **They're little chemical messengers that zip around, telling your cells what to do, when to do it, and how much of it needs to be done.** Like getting an emoji-filled text from a friend that says, "Party at my place!" Your cells jump into action, just like you would, pulling on your party shoes.

Now, where do these hormones come from? Think of hormone-producing glands like tiny, specialized factories in your body.

Some of the big players are the **pituitary gland**, the **thyroid**, and the **adrenal glands**, among others. Each factory specializes in making certain types of hormones, and they're really good at it!

Imagine a "mood factory" churning out serotonin and dopamine, while another "growth factory" is busy making hormones that help you grow tall or build muscles.

The creation of hormones is a fascinating blend of science and magic - well, biochemistry, to be exact!

Let's say the brain senses that you need more energy because you're running a marathon. It sends a signal to the adrenal glands, like hitting the "emergency" button, and voila! They produce adrenaline, your body's very own "turbo-charge," giving you that extra oomph to cross the finish line.

So, what sort of shenanigans do hormones get up to once they're in action? Well, they have a say in just about everything! Need to grow? Hormones. Need to sleep? Hormones. Feeling stressed, happy, or hungry? Yep, you guessed it - hormones! From regulating your heartbeat to helping you digest that delicious burrito, hormones are the unsung heroes behind the scenes.

But what happens if our hormonal messengers get their signals crossed?

That's when things can go haywire. Too much or too little of a hormone can result in various conditions, like insomnia, weight gain, or even mood swings.

Think of it as sending too many emojis in a text; the message can get confusing! That's why the delicate balance of hormones is so crucial, and understanding them can be a key to unlocking optimal health.

So there you have it!

Hormones are your body's multitasking messengers, taking care of everything from your mood to your metabolism. Created in specialized "factories," they zip around the bloodstream, delivering vital messages to keep you functioning at your best. They're like the backstage crew of a big production—out of sight, but making sure the show goes on without a hitch!

You can also think of hormones as the body's ultimate communication system, akin to text messages sprinkled with emojis and GIFs.

These tiny molecules are chemical messengers that have the power to alter cell behavior and orchestrate complex bodily functions. Imagine a flurry of emojis: tells your body it's time to sleep, while signals energy and movement. Just like how you'd interpret these emojis and adjust your actions accordingly, hormones guide your cells to act in specific ways, whether it's to rev up your metabolism or calm down your stress levels.

Now, where do these hormones originate?

Picture specialized glands throughout your body as miniature factories, each with its own production specialty. We've got the thyroid gland acting like the energy manager, cranking out hormones that control metabolic rate.

Imagine it as your body's power plant, making sure you have enough juice to get through the day.

Then there's the adrenal gland, the stress and fight-or-flight headquarters. When you encounter a bear while hiking—or more realistically, a mountain of emails—your adrenal glands churn out cortisol and adrenaline like a dedicated barista during morning rush hour.

How do these factories know when to start production? It all begins with a stimulus. Let's say you're running late for an important meeting; your brain senses the urgency and sends a signal to your adrenal glands.

It's like someone pushing a big red button labeled *"EMERGENCY"* in a control room.

Boom! Your adrenal glands get the memo and start creating adrenaline, giving you that surge of energy to dash to your meeting like you're competing in the Olympics.

Once these hormones are manufactured, think of them as tiny cruise ships embarking on a voyage through the bloodstream. They drift along until they find their target port - a specific cell or organ that's wired to receive their message.

Each hormone has a unique "docking station," known as a receptor, where it unloads its message like a postman delivering mail. For example, insulin, the sugar regulator, docks onto cells and essentially says, ***"Hey, open up! We've got some sugar that needs storing!"***

When the cells get the message, they obediently open up, pulling sugar from the blood to store or use.

Now, ***hormones are not lone rangers***; they usually work in complex networks, like a group of friends planning a weekend getaway. Each one has a specific role, and they need to coordinate for everything to go smoothly.

The thyroid hormones and the pituitary gland, for instance, are like the ***"planners"*** in your friend group. The pituitary gland keeps tabs on thyroid levels and, if they dip, sends out TSH (Thyroid Stimulating Hormone) as if texting, "Hey, we need more energy here. Fire up the grills!"

Life events like puberty, pregnancy, and menopause can drastically change your hormonal landscape.

Imagine a switchboard lighting up with new connections and rerouting old ones. It's as if your body got a software update and is adapting to the changes by balancing a cocktail of hormones like estrogen, progesterone, and testosterone. During puberty, for example, estrogen and testosterone are like the party planners announcing, ***"Surprise! Welcome to adulthood, here are some new features for you to explore."***

Hormonal imbalances can lead to a cascade of issues—picture a symphony orchestra out of tune. Maybe your sleep cycle is disrupted, or you're always feeling anxious. Diagnosing hormonal issues often involves blood tests, as hormones leave a detectable trace. It's like doing a roll call to see who's missing or who's being too loud in the orchestra. Once identified, hormonal imbalances can often be managed with medication, lifestyle changes, or even hormone replacement therapies, getting you back to your harmonious symphony of well-being.

So there you have it, a detailed yet entertaining look into the dynamic world of hormones! They're like the maestros conducting the orchestra that is your body, making sure every instrument (or in this case, cell and organ) plays its part in the grand performance of life.

So now that we've toured the "Hormone Symphony Orchestra," how about a little peek at the "VIP lineup?" Think of it as the music festival lineup card, where each artist - or in this case, hormone - has its unique act and role to play in keeping you awesome. Ready to meet some of the headliners?

Let's dive into a table that showcases what these superstar hormones do!

Hormone	What It Does & Fun Facts
Estrogen	The "Girly Gear" hormone! It kickstarts puberty in females, oversees the menstrual cycle, and is the go - to hormone for libido, breast health, and all things feminine.
Progesterone	The "Balancer." Takes care of menstrual cycle, mood, sleep and even appetite. It's your wellness BFF!
FSH	"Start me up!" Makes the menstrual cycle hit the road. It's a **MUST CHECK** blood marker for those entering menopause.
LH	The "Go Signal." Triggers ovulation and makes testosterone in guys. Basically, LH is the "starting whistle" for reproductive races.
Insulin	"Sugar Cop." Regulates blood sugar by storing it away. But watch out - if it hangs around too long, you may pack on the pounds!

Hormone	What It Does & Fun Facts
Glucagon	The "Lifesaver." It raises your blood sugar when it becomes alarmingly low. It's like the backup generator for your body.
Testosterone	The "Manly Maker." It does everything from building muscles to regulating libido. ***Yes, ladies have it too.***
Thyroxin (T4)	The "Tuner." It regulates everything from metabolism to body temperature.
TSH	"The conductor." TSH comes from the brain to tell the thyroid to get to work. This hormone calls a lot of the shots.
Anti-diuretic Hormone	"Water Keeper." This hormone helps your body hold on to water and keeps blood pressure in check.
Ghrelin	Think, "Hunger Games." This hormone stimulates your appetite and is highly regulated by sleep. It's your stomach's SOS.
Leptin	"The Satisfier." Leptin signals when you're full and regulates energy. It's the stop sign at the end of your meal.
Melatonin	"Nighty night." Melatonin kicks in when it gets dark to help you catch those ZZZ's.

> ***Did you know you are a walking, talking, shopping bunch of hormones?***
>
> ***Hormones control everything we are and do!***

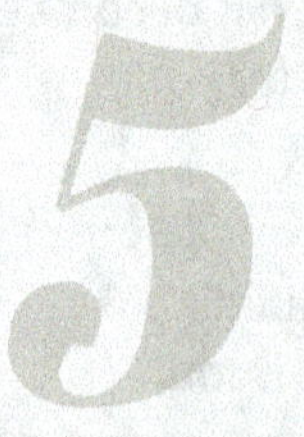

Chapter 5

UNDERSTANDING YIN AND YANG OF HORMONES

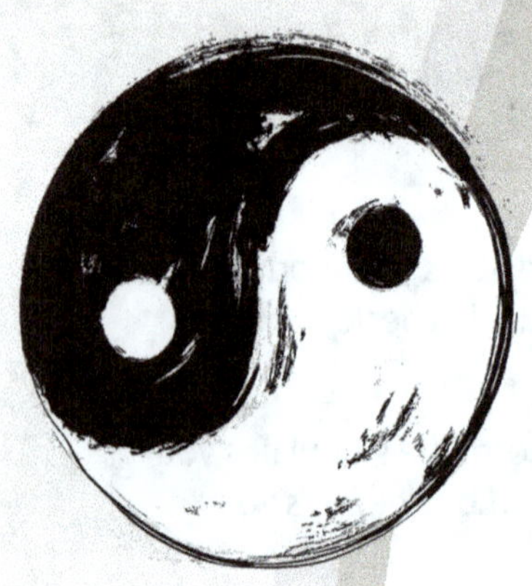

Our bodies are always striving for equilibrium, like two dance partners who know their moves down to a tee.

Hormones are the ultimate Yin and Yang, always in sync, always conversing like lifelong best friends. Just like the ancient Chinese philosophy, they embody the principle that everything - yes, even the universe - is interconnected in a delicate balance.

A Balanced Universe is a Harmonious Universe

This can't be a competition. it's more like a cooperative dance. Harmony is the goal of the universal orchestra conductor, making sure all instruments are in tune. Mess with that, and you're messing with the music of life itself.

Now, we often live in a "more is more" society. But when we embrace balance, we realize that this just isn't the case. Every decision has its pros and cons, the universe's own checks and balances. Accept this, and your body becomes a well-orchestrated symphony.

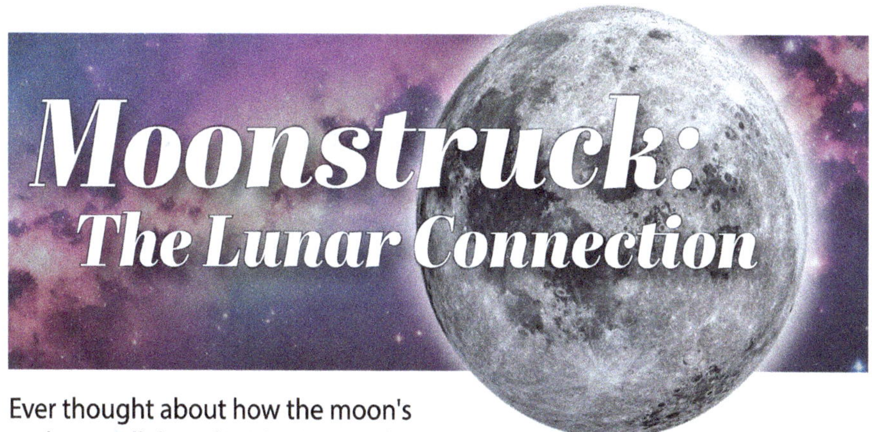

Ever thought about how the moon's cycles parallel our lives? A "normal" menstrual cycle lasts roughly 28 days, which is - surprise, surprise - the same amount of time the moon takes to orbit the Earth.

Coincidence?

Probably not.

Even more fascinating is the **Saros cycle** - every 223 months, or about every nine years, the sun, moon, and moon's nodes align.

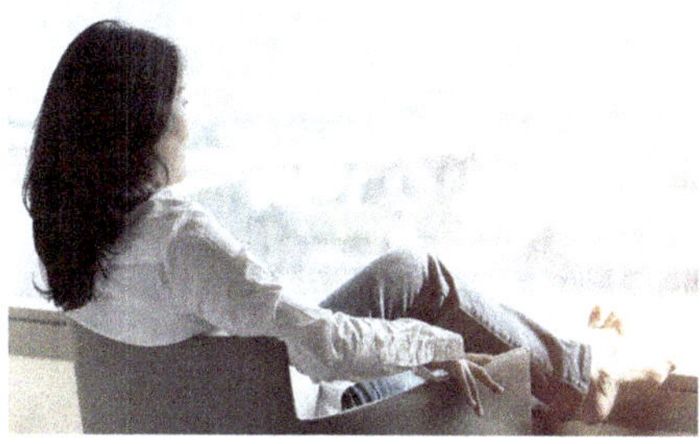

Ever noticed significant life changes happening every nine years? Whether it's the onset of puberty, choosing a career, experiencing a mid-life crisis, or entering menopause, the universe seems to be nudging us along.

When we reject the Yin-Yang balance, we trip up our own metabolic harmony. Sure, we have technology that can mess with this - think pharmaceuticals that throw your hormones off kilter.

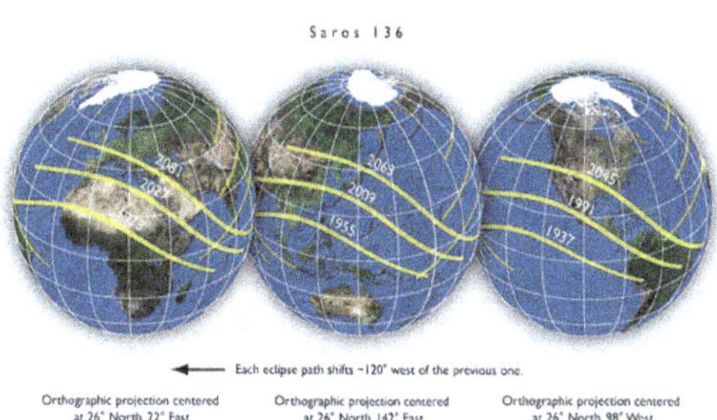

The Saros Cycle = 6585.3 days (18 Years and 10.3 days).

The solar eclipse cycle of about 40 solar eclipses, starts with an eclipse in the polar region each time with 120° farther west (0.3 days).

Let's dive into some examples. Take Progesterone and Estrogen, for instance. They're the classic dynamic duo of hormone science, maintaining a feedback loop that balances each other out like dance partners. If Insulin is the Yin that lowers your blood sugar, then its Yang, Glucagon, brings it back up.

And don't get me started on Thyroid hormones! They find their balance through a feed back system with **TSH**, a hormone produced in the brain.

Even **Leptin** and **Ghrelin**, our hormones of hunger and fullness, join this cosmic dance and **are closely tied to how much sleep we get.**

Some hormones wear multiple hats and have multiple names. Take Growth Hormone, for example. Its counterbalance, Somatostatin, also goes by the intriguing acronym GHIH (Growth Hormone-Inhibiting Hormone) or the long-winded "Somatotropin Release Inhibiting Factor."

Talk about an identity crisis! This hormone's jack-of-all-trades nature helps it regulate many other hormones, ensuring the body stays in a happy equilibrium.

Some hormones are like savvy shoppers; they know how to balance based on what's in stock. Take calcium, for instance. Its hormone bouncer is the Parathyroid Hormone, which helps keep calcium levels steady in the bloodstream. But wait, there's another player! Meet Calcitonin, the yin to Parathyroid Hormone's yang, stepping in to lower calcium levels when needed.

Hormones are the body's cellular messengers. There are two main types: PPAs (Proteins, Peptides, Amino Acids) and Steroid Hormones. PPAs like to chat with cell receptors, sometimes unlocking cellular doors or switching genes on and off like light switches. Steroid hormones, on the other hand, go straight inside the cell to exert their influence.

The term "hormone" actually hails from the Greek word 'horman,' meaning "to urge on" or "impulse." It's like the cheerleader for your body, rooting for specific actions or changes.

The Uber of Hormones?!

Guess what?

You actually need cholesterol. All steroid hormones are made from these fat molecules, and they're like socialites—they don't just show up anywhere. They hop into "hormone taxis," or carrier proteins, to get where they need to go.

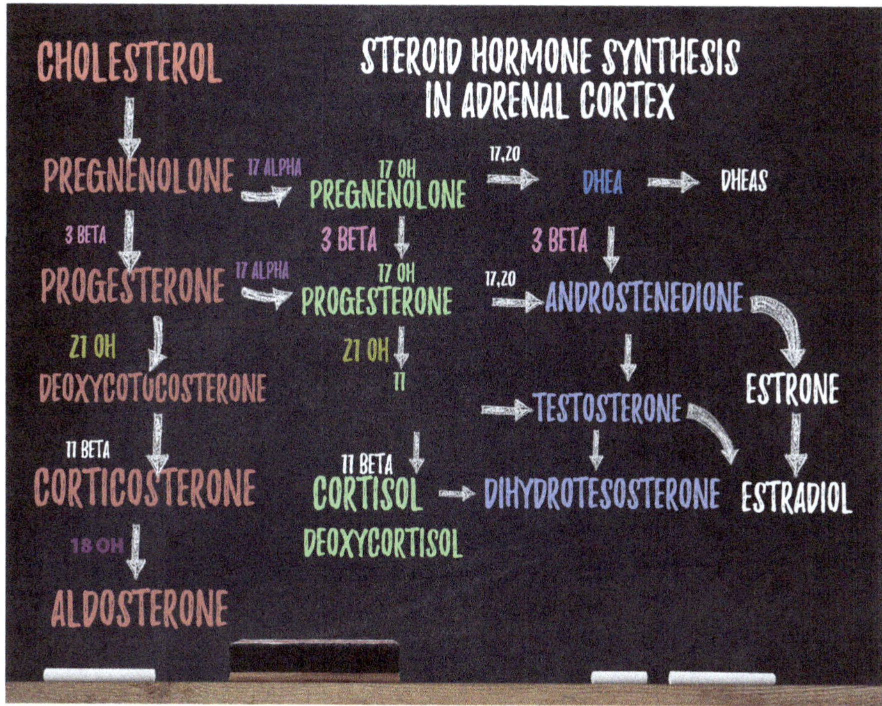

Steroid hormones are sorted into five main groups: glucocorticoids (sugar managers), mineralocorticoids (salt bouncers), androgens (hello, Testosterone), estrogens, and progestogens. Vitamin D is like their cool cousin.

Cholesterol is a molecule that has been vilified for years, often branded as the bad guy waiting in the shadows to ambush your arteries. But let's set the record straight: cholesterol isn't just a fat globule cruising through your bloodstream, waiting to trigger a heart attack. **Far from it!**

Think of cholesterol as the building block, or the raw material, in your body's hormone factory. It's the essential "ingredient" that your body uses to whip up a batch of vital hormones, like estrogen, testosterone, and even Vitamin D.

Yes, without cholesterol, your body's hormone balance would be like a see-saw with only one side - lopsided and dysfunctional.

But the story doesn't end with hormones. Did you know that **Vitamin D, a hormone-like substance made from cholesterol**, plays a key role in calcium absorption?

Yup!

So, if you're low on cholesterol, your bones might just feel the brunt of it. And let's face it, nobody wants to be hunched over like the Hunchback of Notre Dame in their golden years!

Your brain is a fatty organ—about %60 fat, to be exact—and cholesterol is one of its main components. So, you could say that cholesterol is the brain's BFF, helping with everything from neurotransmitter function to keeping those synapses firing at full speed.

If cholesterol were a student, it would be the class valedictorian of Brain Health High!

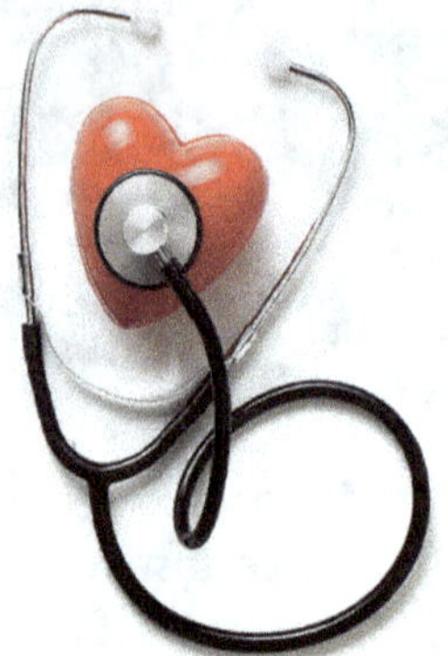

Now, here's where it gets interesting. Contrary to popular belief, cholesterol is not the sole villain in the heart health narrative. It actually plays a crucial role in cellular repair, and guess what? Your heart is a big bundle of cells! While it's true that excessive LDL ("bad" cholesterol) levels can be harmful, it's all about balance. Your body also produces HDL ("good" cholesterol) to keep things in check. It's the yin and yang of cardiovascular wellness.

So, next time someone mentions cholesterol, don't imagine a fatty blob lurking in your arteries. Instead, picture a busy worker bee, buzzing around to make sure your hormones, bones, brain, and even your heart are all in tip-top shape!

That's enough science jargon for now! These basics help us understand why hormonal balance isn't just good—it's essential!

The pursuit of balance is a lifelong journey, especially when it comes to hormones. My commitment to this field isn't just professional; it's deeply personal. I've seen firsthand the transformative power of natural bioidentical hormones, not only in my life but also in the lives of countless women I've had the privilege to treat.

Let's be real: Medical schools and residency programs don't cover this stuff. That's why I took it upon myself to learn from the pioneers in the field. Over the years, I've refined my approach, always aiming for that sweet spot of hormonal equilibrium for each individual.

Life has an interesting way of setting us on paths we never intended to walk. For me, that path was laden with hurdles that forced me to reckon with my own body.

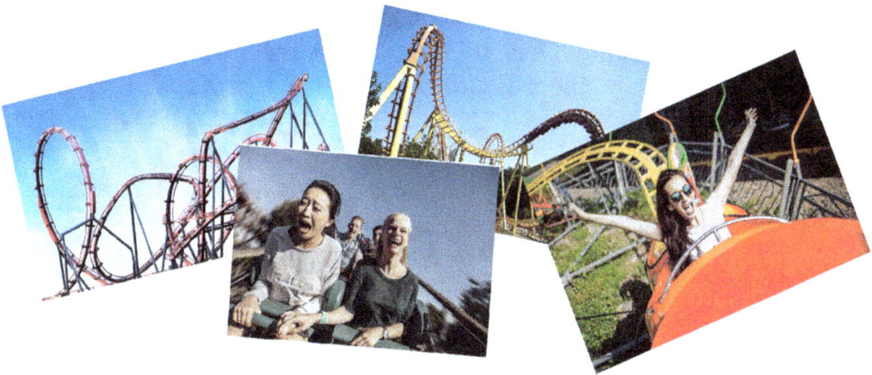

Yes, you read that right. It is quite the list.

The conventional solutions, especially synthetic hormones, only intensified the storm inside me. Think of putting diesel fuel into a gasoline engine; things just got worse. It was like my body was waving red flags, forcing me to pay attention.

I've always believed that the universe, or God, or whatever higher power you subscribe to, doesn't throw curveballs at us to mess with us, but to point us in a direction.

For me, these challenges were not stumbling blocks but stepping stones, pushing me to venture outside the box and dig deeper. It was as if life handed me a toolkit, albeit a challenging one, and said, "Here, figure this out. There's treasure at the end."

So, I took that toolkit and made it my mission to learn everything I could. I took on the role of the student, devouring wisdom from the visionaries in the field and marrying that knowledge with my own clinical experiences. The more I uncovered, the more I realized that my struggles weren't just my own; they were a window into the world of so many others grappling with similar issues.

The beauty of this journey? It's been a two-way street. While it felt like these and marrying that knowledge with my own clinical experiences. The more I uncovered, the more I realized that my struggles weren't just my own; they were a window into the world of so many others grappling with similar issues.

The beauty of this journey? It's been a two-way street. While it felt like these challenges were "done to me," I now see that they were, in fact, done for me and by extension, for my patients. My struggles became the key that unlocked new possibilities for countless individuals. Think of it as turning lemons into the most therapeutic lemonade you could imagine.

As I healed myself, I became better equipped to guide others towards their own healing. It's been an incredibly rewarding cycle, one where the teacher becomes the student and vice versa. Also, while it's easy to see challenges as burdens, I now understand them as *gifts*, wrapped in layers of complexity, but gifts nonetheless.

In the grand tapestry of life, it's often the snags that make the most interesting patterns. My health challenges were the snags in my tapestry, and as I navigated through each one, not only did I enrich my own life but I was able to turn those threads into lifelines for my patients. And for that, I wouldn't change a thing.

Among the things I discovered that changed everything (there would be many amazing things to add to our clinic's arsenal of Regenerative and Integrative medicine, but let's not get ahead of ourselves) were the advances in Bio-identical hormone production and the incredible results from their application.

So, what are Bio-identical hormone?

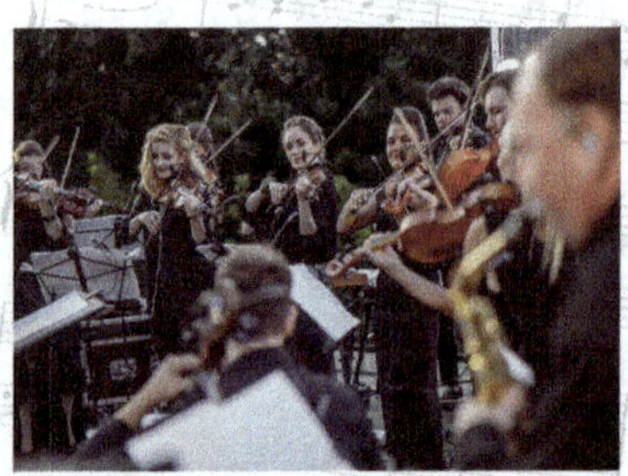

Again, imagine your body as a finely tuned orchestra, with each instrument (or   hormone, in our case) playing a vital role. Bio-identical hormones are like the   original sheet music, matching the body's natural hormones note-for-note.

Starring the HPA Axis (Hypothalamus-Pituitary-Adrenal) as the conductor. Each hormone is a different instrument, playing its part in the symphony of your body. When one is out of tune, the whole ensemble suffers. The real maestro in this musical analogy is stress, directing the hormones in their various roles, for better or for worse.

Now, think of synthetic hormones as cover bands. They play the same tunes but with a different vibe, and sometimes the audience (your body) doesn't react well to these altered compositions.

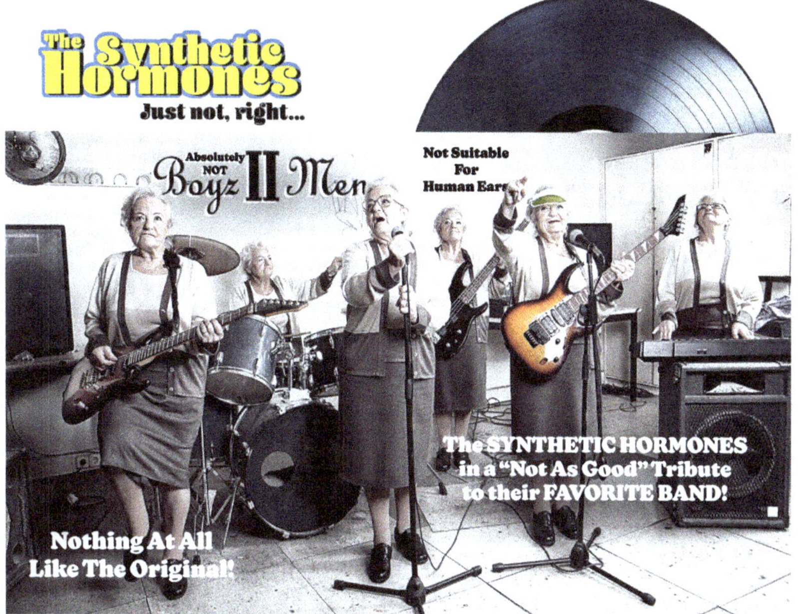

Synthetic hormones may have similar effects, but their molecular structure doesn't quite match our natural hormones. This slight discord can lead to a range of symptoms and possible side effects.

Enter the world of compounding - or, the art of making personalized medications. It's like having a personal chef who knows exactly how you like your meals. Compounding allows us to create a 'custom cocktail' of hormones tailored to each person's unique needs, as revealed by their lab tests and symptoms.

This leads to a "one size fits all," versus a "custom fit" model for these valuable medicines. Commercially available bio-identical hormones like estradiol and progesterone are great, but they come in standard doses.

That's like buying a one-size-fits-all shirt; it might fit, but maybe not perfectly.

On the other hand, compounded bio-identical hormones are customized to fit you like a glove, or in this case, match your unique hormonal profile.

Let's say your body is like a unique musical composition, a symphony that requires different notes or 'hormone levels' to perform optimally.

Traditional dosing methods would be like a music teacher handing you a standard sheet of music, ignoring your unique style. Compounded bio-identical hormones are like having a composer write a symphony just for you.

Here's the cherry on top. With compounded bio-identical hormones, you're not stuck with just one form of delivery. It's like choosing between takeout, home-cooked meals, or fine dining. You can get your hormones in creams, troches (lozenges), or even patches, which may not always be an option with commercial pharmaceuticals.

In a nutshell, bio-identical hormones give us the tools to create a harmonious balance that's as unique as you are. By tailoring your treatment based on specialized labs and your personal experience, we get closer to hitting that perfect note in your life's symphony.

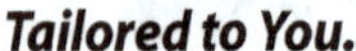

Tailored to You.

This customization is based on lab tests like saliva or blood work, but mostly by how you're feeling — your symptoms or concerns. And not everyone needs hormone therapy; some might find balance through nutrition and lifestyle changes alone. However, when hormonal supplements are needed, bioidentical ones are often the safer choice.

Periodic testing is essential. Think of it as your hormonal 'state of the union' address. It allows your healthcare provider to fine-tune your treatment and rule out underlying issues like tumors.
A Note on Synthetic Hormones

We've all heard the cautionary tales, especially from studies like the Women's Health Initiative (WHI). But remember, those studies focused on synthetic hormones. Their findings don't necessarily apply to bioidentical hormones, when done correctly.

Nothing is done without risk. Hormones are tricky and should be managed by a medical professional that really knows what they are doing.

Hormonal balance isn't just about alleviating symptoms; i***t's about integrative and functional medicine well-being.*** From osteoporosis prevention to maintaining youthful skin and mental agility, the benefits are manifold.

The controversy surrounding hormone replacement therapy (HRT) and cancer is real. So much so that many doctors shy away from prescribing any form of HRT to women with a history of breast cancer.

For a deeper dive into this topic, I highly recommend Dr. John Lee's book, "What Your Doctor May Not Tell You About Breast Cancer," among his other works. These books are my go-to   resources for hormone education.

I would be remiss in not giving tribute to Dr. Lee, as he impacted every aspect of hormone management that I carry today with my patients.

Dr. John R. Lee was a trailblazer, the kind of pioneer who looked beyond the conventional wisdom of his time. Imagine him as the first artist in a new genre of music, introducing fresh rhythms and melodies that nobody had heard before. He was the one who popularized the term **"bio-identical hormones"** and made it mainstream, much like a hit song that everyone suddenly can't stop humming.

Dr. Lee was a family physician who turned into a hormone superstar. Frustrated with the 'one-size-fits-all' approach of synthetic hormone replacement therapy (HRT), he explored alternative paths and ultimately became an advocate for natural, bio-identical hormones.

He's the kind of doctor who didn't just keep his discoveries to himself but shared them through books and articles. His works, like "What Your Doctor May Not Tell You About Menopause," became bestsellers and are considered seminal texts in the world of hormone health. Think of these books as the "classical compositions" that many hormone experts, like myself, still refer to as their 'bibles.'

Dr. Lee coined the term **"estrogen dominance"** to describe the condition where a person has an imbalance of estrogen relative to progesterone, setting the stage for many hormonal-related issues. ***That's like recognizing a new genre of music that others were hesitant to acknowledge.***

Although Dr. Lee is no longer with us, his work laid the foundation for further studies and gave credibility to the use of bio-identical hormones. Like a legendary musician whose songs continue to inspire, his contributions to medicine continue to help countless individuals find balance and health in their lives.

In many ways, Dr. John Lee is to bio-identical hormones what Elvis is to rock 'n' roll - an unforgettable pioneer who changed the game forever.

A key take-away, from these works would definitely be that hormonal balance can be a complex journey involving more than a casual level of committment and adherence.

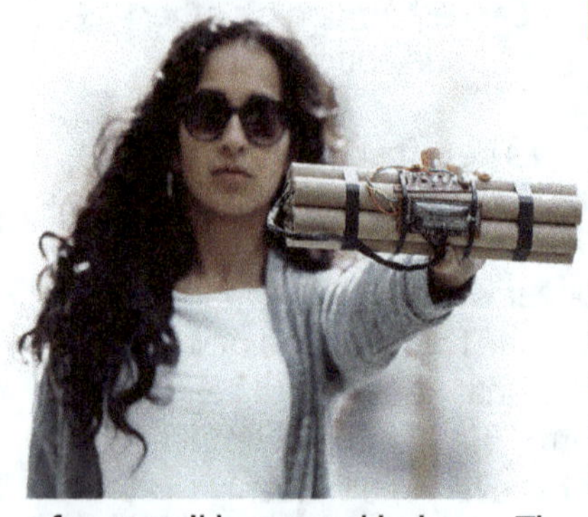

NOT ALL ESTROGENS ARE BAD.

Estrogen often gets villainized, largely thanks to a 2002 study that sowed fear and confusion about hormone therapy. This study had three main flaws: it used synthetic hormones, employed an ineffective and potentially dangerous delivery method, and ignored the necessity for overall hormonal balance. These are   pitfalls that I work diligently to avoid in my own protocols.

Premenopausal women produce three key types of estrogen:

estrone (E1)

estradiol (E2)

estriol (E3)

While estrone and estradiol are potent, estriol is considered a weaker estrogen. There's a theory that estrone is the "bad guy" linked to cancer, while estriol might be cancer-protective. Estradiol seems to be neutral in this equation.

Let's dig into the estrogen trio: estrone (E1), estradiol (E2), and estriol (E3).

Think of these three estrogens like the Goldilocks story - each one has its own **"just right"** scenario, but they can wreak havoc when they're out of balance.

Estrone (E1): Sometimes called the "storage estrogen," this one is mostly produced by fat cells. Imagine it like the long-lasting battery in your remote control. It's always there, even when you're not using it. **Estrone has been a subject of concern because it's thought to be a more "aggressive" form of estrogen, often linked to certain types of cancers, including breast cancer.**

Estradiol (E2): This is the diva of the estrogen world, the one responsible for all the glitz and glamour of femininity—smooth skin, robust hair, and reproductive health. It's your body's main estrogen during your reproductive years. Picture it as the high-powered fuel in a race car; **it does the heavy lifting but needs to be in just the right amount.**

Estriol (E3): Often called the "forgotten" estrogen, this one is considered the kindest, gentler form. It's the major estrogen during pregnancy but is often present in smaller amounts during other phases of life. ***Think of estriol as the soft, dim light that creates ambiance but isn't going to blind you if you stare at it. It's considered a "protector" estrogen because of its weaker and potentially anti-cancer properties.***

The theory about estrone being the "bad guy" comes from its association with certain cancers, while estriol might be the "guardian angel," stepping in to mitigate some of those risks. Estradiol is like the neutral judge, playing an essential but balanced role.

How these estrogens interact is key. It's not just about one being "bad" and another being "good," it's about how they all work in harmony, like an orchestra. If one section drowns out the others, you don't get beautiful music—you get noise.

So, first, let's talk about estriol (E3). *This is a fascinating estrogen because it's kind of like the security guard at a nightclub, monitoring who comes in and who doesn't.* In this case, the "nightclub" is the estrogen receptor on breast tissue cells.

Estriol has a weaker affinity for these receptors, but by occupying them, it blocks the more potent, aggressive estrone (E1) from taking that spot and promoting cell proliferation, which could be a potential setup for cancer.

It's almost like estriol is the soft-spoken family member at Thanksgiving dinner who brings balance to the table, while estrone is the loud, boisterous relative who could cause a scene if not moderated. And guess what? Many doctors are completely unaware of this protective bouncer-like role estriol can play.

It's a vital piece of the puzzle that can be lifesaving, especially for women with a family history of breast cancer.

As for estrone (E1), you hit the nail on the head. It's fantastic if you're nine years old and need to develop breast tissue, but for a menopausal woman, it's like bringing a flame thrower to a candlelit dinner - way too much and potentially disastrous.

The ego clash with mainstream doctors can be a frustrating maze to navigate. I had a patient with a strong family history of breast cancer who saw a specialist - one who, of all people, should have been in the know.

The specialist had to Google this vital information during the consultation! Can you imagine?

The term "estrogen" is tossed around like it's a single entity, but it's misleading. What we should be saying is "estrogens," plural, because the different types come with different roles and risks. It's like saying "fruit" when what you really mean is oranges, apples, and grapes—all of which have distinct nutritional profiles.

Let's consider the estrogen paradox: If all "estrogen" were bad, then wouldn't nine-year-old girls have a high risk of breast cancer, given their estrone levels? *The key is balance! It's about the orchestra of E1, E2, and E3 playing in harmony.* When this musical trio is out of sync, that's when health issues arise.

The ratio of estrone to estriol is a critical indicator, and let's not forget estradiol's (E2) role as the referee, especially after menopause when its levels drop, disrupting the balance and potentially increasing the risk of various diseases.

So yes, *knowing your estrogen levels and strategically supplementing, especially with protective estriol, could literally be a life-saving strategy.*

Makes sense, doesn't it?

So, in the journey for optimal health, especially when it comes to hormone replacement therapy, the goal is to get these three estrogens to play their most beautiful symphony.

The route of administering estrogens matters. Oral estrogens go through the liver, getting converted to estrone, which can potentially have negative effects. In contrast, systemic routes (like patches, creams, or under-the-tongue applications) bypass this liver metabolism.

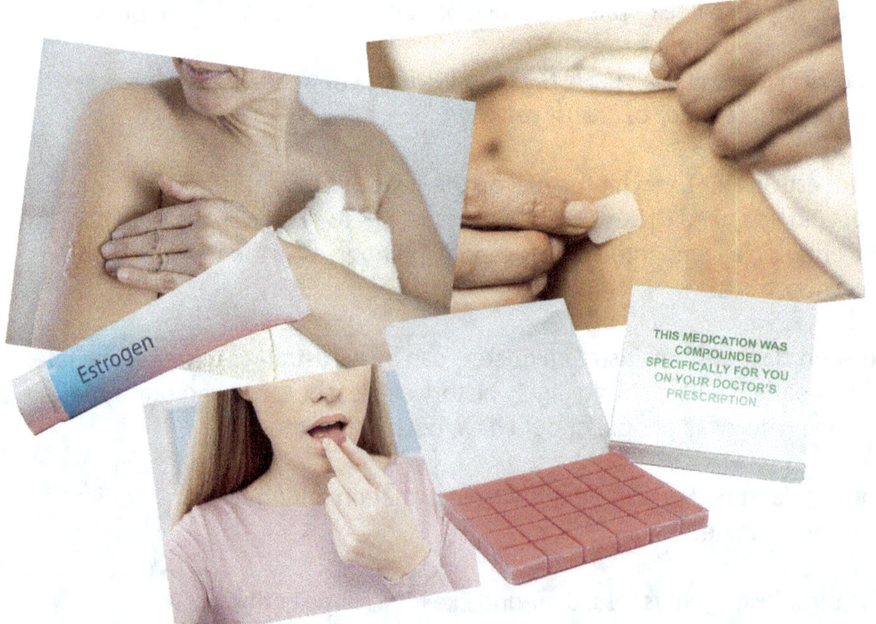

its focus on postmenopausal women when HRT is often used for perimeno-pausal symptoms. Even if the absolute risks are small, the relative risks, such as the increase in heart attacks or breast cancer, can be significant.

Thankfully, better options exist. Dr. John Lee, a pioneer in bioidentical hor-mone therapy, proposed three rules: use hormones only if needed, opt for bi-oidentical over synthetic, and aim for hormonal balance. Sometimes, all that's needed for symptom control is proper nutritional and endocrine support.

Switching from synthetic to bioidentical hormones can be a transition. Hor-mone receptors accustomed to synthetic molecules may take time to adapt. A gradual shift, rather than going "cold turkey," helps to mitigate flare-ups of symptoms like hot flashes.

I had a patient with a family history of breast cancer consult a breast cancer specialist, who—believe it or not—had to Google this vital information in the examination room. This knowledge gap is alarming and a perfect example of the dangers of not individualizing hormone treatment plans.

"How Long will I need to be on Hormone therapy?"

The answer to this depends on how long you have symptoms or the body has issues consistent with hormone deficiencies. For some this is a few months, for others many years. When your body is in balance your adrenal glands can make all the same hormones that your ovaries can, so adrenal health is very important if a patient wants to get off any type of supplemental hormone therapy.

I have also come to learn about "leaky gut and nutrition", that all hormone im-balance starts in the gut so if you address and repair those issues while giving attention to any other hormone imbalance like adrenal or thyroid issues then you won't need hormone supplementation.

Your body can make and regulate hormones perfectly if the conditions are right. ***EVEN after a total hysterectomy!***

I also get asked about having periods after menopause.

It is not necessary for a postmenopausal woman to have periods if using   bi-oidentical hormones properly. When postmenopausal women use small doses of bioidentical hormones, they rarely, if ever, have periods.

I also get asked about having periods after menopause. It is not necessary for a postmenopausal woman to have periods if using bioidentical hormones properly. *When postmenopausal women use small doses of bioidentical hormones, they rarely, if ever, have periods.* Nor do they have the risky endometrial buildup in the uterus which is what makes it important to have periods.

Estrogen stimulates the buildup of uterine tissue, but there's no need to take that much estrogen to feel healthy and balanced. *Since fat cells create estrogen, women who are heavy may not even need to use supplemental estrogen.*

Dr. Lee's recommendation was always to use the lowest dose possible of any hormone supplementation. Usually this was 15 to 30 mg of progesterone daily, and the lowest dose of estrogen that would either clear up estrogen deficiency symptoms or show normal levels on a saliva hormone level test. This improves health and well-being, but doesn't put a postmenopausal woman back into the same hormonal milieu I had when I was menstruating every month.

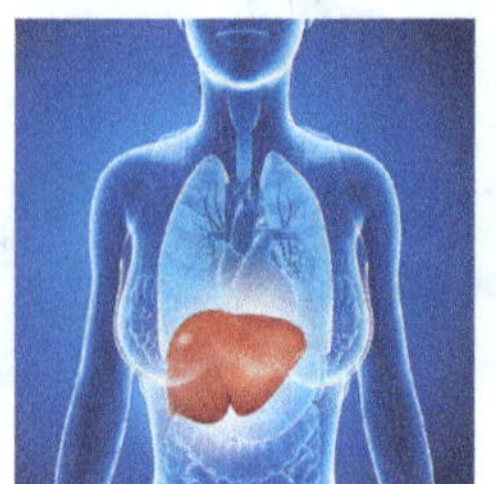

When you take progesterone in a pill form, most of it goes directly to the liver, where up to 70 percent of it may be dumped, but not before creating a variety of byproducts (metabolites).

Thus, it's necessary to take 100 mg of progesterone in pill form to get 20 mg into your cells.

If your liver happens to be working less efficiently on a given day, and excretes less of the progesterone, it's easy to experience overdose side effects, such as sleepiness and bloating.

These side effects often have women running for more estrogen to wake themselves up again.

What they really need to do is use progesterone cream, which is a much more efficient delivery method.

If you put 20 mg on your skin, virtually all of that will be in your bloodstream within a matter of minutes.

Hormone therapy, along with frequent testing and symptom management, can be a powerful tool in avoiding the nursing home and mitigating the effects of aging.

In the context of aging, hormone imbalances can fast-track us down the road to numerous health issues: Alzheimer's, weakened bones that can easily fracture, incontinence, and accelerated skin aging, to name a few.

Maintaining hormonal balance is akin to optimizing the performance of this "bodily orchestra." By doing so, we're not just controlling symptoms; we're managing the root cause, helping the body to function as optimally as possible.

It's not just about estrogen. The hormonal spectrum is vast, including but not limited to insulin, thyroid, and adrenal hormones. These hormones collectively contribute to how quickly we age and how well we age.

It's much like maintaining a car. You wouldn't just focus on keeping the engine oil clean while ignoring the brakes, would you? Every part has its role, and neglecting one can lead to a cascade of problems. Similarly, even if estrogen isn't in the picture, there are still a plethora of other "parts" or hormones that need attention.

Big Pharma, unfortunately has an agenda that benefits from wanting to keep the spotlight away from this approach. The pharmaceutical industry often aims to treat the symptom and not the cause. ***A headache is not an aspirin deficiency.*** We've got to look beyond just putting on Band-Aids on the issues and aim for a comprehensive, systemic approach that addresses the root causes.

And here's where the beauty of what I, and so many experts who are passionate in this field do, comes in, we share about alternative routes; creating alternative pathways for people to follow.

That's not just medicine; that's life-changing advocacy. I have seen over 30,000 patients in my 24 plus years of clinical practice and feel confident in every patient that I see that I am making a difference and that feeds my heart and soul. I don't say that to impress you but to impress upon you that many people have found this path and ***you deserve to feel, look and be the best you possible!***

I didn't intend to embark on this journey. It seems to have found me, but I'm so grateful it did.

How long will I take bio-identical hormones… I think you know now!

Notes...

Chapter 6

Hormone Testing

Hormone testing is a cornerstone of understanding what's going on in the body and how best to balance it.

Let's think of hormone testing as taking a "snapshot" of your body's internal communication system.

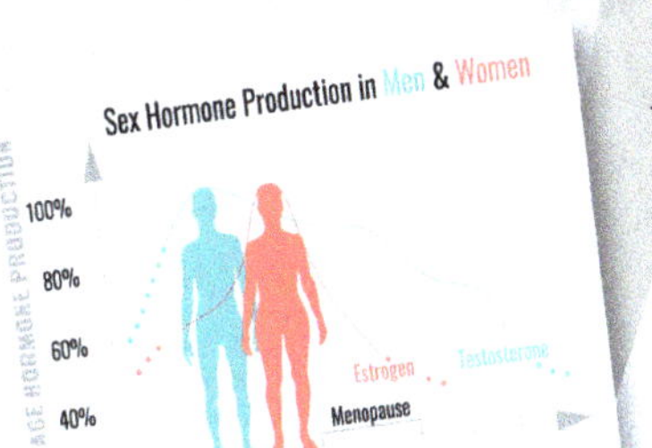

Here's a table to break down the essentials, but this is by no means a comprehensive list. Just for a few examples, I have broken some down in a table to help you understand a groundwork for your advocacy.

ESTROGEN Think of these as the Yin and Yang of female reproductive health. You need to know both to understand the full picture of what's going on.	**PREGNENOLONE** Think of this as the "parent" molecule to many other hormones. If it's imbalanced, the "kids" may act out.
TESTOSTERONE Yes, women have it too, and it's crucial for energy and drive!	**FSH & LH** These are the messengers that tell your ovaries what to do each month. If the message isn't clear, things like fertility and menstrual cycles go haywire.
DHEA & CORTISOL Your adrenal glands make these, and if they're out of whack, it's like trying to drive a car with a flat tire.	**IGF-1** This is like your body's internal fountain of youth, and it can affect how quickly you age.
THYROID HORMONES Think of your thyroid as your body's thermostat. Too high or too low, and you're going to feel it.	**MELATONIN** Like your internal alarm clock, this hormone tells you when it's time to hit the sack.
INSULIN This is like your body's accountant, keeping track of the energy (sugar) you're taking in. Get this wrong, and you risk being "audited" by diabetes.	*Testing these hormones provides a comprehensive view, like looking at the weather report for every season. If you know what to expect, you can prepare accordingly and make better health decision.*

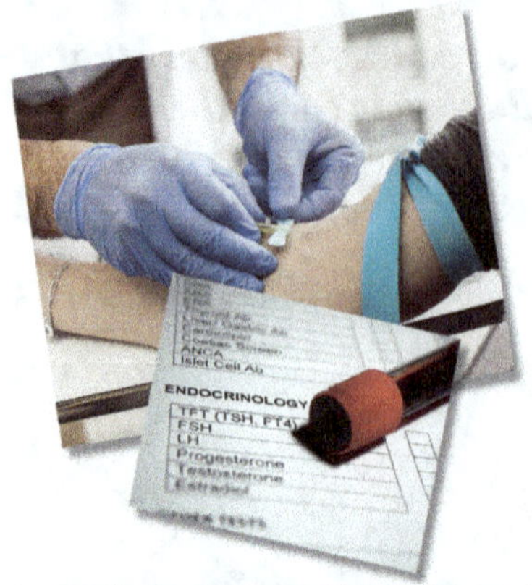

HOW SHOULD I GET TESTED?

So you're ready to get the inside scoop on your hormones?

Fantastic!

Just like you'd check under the hood if your car starts making funny noises, it's time to check your hormone levels when you notice symptoms.

I usually recommend a full panel to get the most accurate "snapshot" of your hormonal landscape. This isn't just limited to ovarian hormones like estrogens (estrone, estradiol, estriol), progesterone, and testosterone. We should also peek at adrenal and thyroid hormones, along with more specific tests if your symptoms point that way.

Think of this as casting a wide net.

you never know what you might catch!

Saliva testing has become a crowd favorite, and for good reason.

Imagine your hormones are like Wi-Fi signals, buzzing around in the air but also through the walls (your tissues). Saliva tests capture these 'through the wall' signals, giving us a more accurate picture of how much is actually reaching the cells.

Though your insurance might give it the side-eye, saliva tests can often be more budget-friendly than their blood test counterparts.

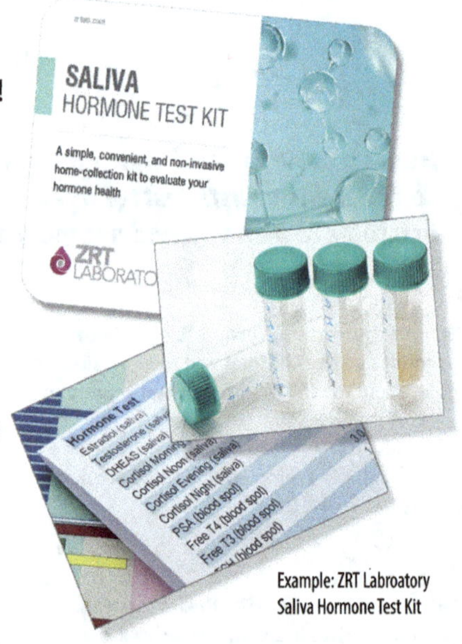

Example: ZRT Labroatory Saliva Hormone Test Kit

Studies have shown that the hormone levels in saliva are a mirror reflection of the 'bio-available' hormones in your blood - those active, "get things done," kind of hormones. Think of it like the "A-team" that's actually out on the field, not just sitting on the bench.

Saliva can capture metrics on several heavy hitters like **estradiol, estrone, estriol, progesterone, testosterone, DHEA-S, and cortisol.**

Saliva testing offers flexibility and convenience. You can do it anywhere, anytime. Imagine trying to catch a beautiful sunrise you have to be there at the right moment.

The same goes for some hormone levels, which are best captured at specific times of the day. And no worries if you're a globe-trotter or a homebody; these samples are sturdy and can be stored at room temperature for a week without losing their mojo.

Personalized Approach

Each of us is as unique as a snowflake, and our hormone profiles are no different. The art lies in aligning this unique hormonal "painting" with your symptoms and lifestyle. As a practitioner, it's like being both a detective and an artist, piecing together the clues to create a balanced, vibrant picture of health.

Blood Serum Testing: Your Comprehensive Health Blueprint

Unlike saliva testing, blood serum tests allow us to peek into a wider range of indicators that go beyond just hormonal balance. It's like upgrading from a basic cable package to premium—more channels, more information!

What Can It Reveal?

Thyroid Hormones:
Think of these as the Yin and Yang of female reproductive health. You need to know both to understand the full picture of what's going on.

Insulin Levels:
Yes, women have it too, and it's crucial for energy and drive!

Vitamin D:
Your adrenal glands make these, and if they're out of whack, it's like trying to drive a car with a flat tire.

Different Estrogens (E1, E2, E3):
Think of your thyroid as your body's thermostat. Too high or too low, and you're going to feel it.

Iron Levels
This is like your body's accountant, keeping track of the energy (sugar) you're taking in. Get this wrong, and you risk being "audited" by diabetes.

CBC (Complete Blood Count):
Think of this as the "parent" molecule to many other hormones. If it's imbalanced, the "kids" may act out.

CMP (Comprehensive Metabolic Panel):
These are the messengers that tell your ovaries what to do each month. If the message isn't clear, things like fertility and menstrual cycles go haywire.

Think of each test as a brushstroke in a painting.

Alone, it might not tell you much, but together they create a comprehensive portrait of you.

Your hormone levels, vitamin deficiencies, organ function - each adds a layer of depth and detail to your health profile.

And here's the kicker: By correlating these blood test results with symptoms, we can really fine-tune your treatment plan. It's like adjusting the color balance, contrast, and saturation in a photograph until it's just perfect.

So while saliva testing is like a quick selfie of your current hormonal state, blood serum testing is the formal portrait that goes into much greater detail.

The two can work in tandem to give you the clearest picture of your health from all angles.

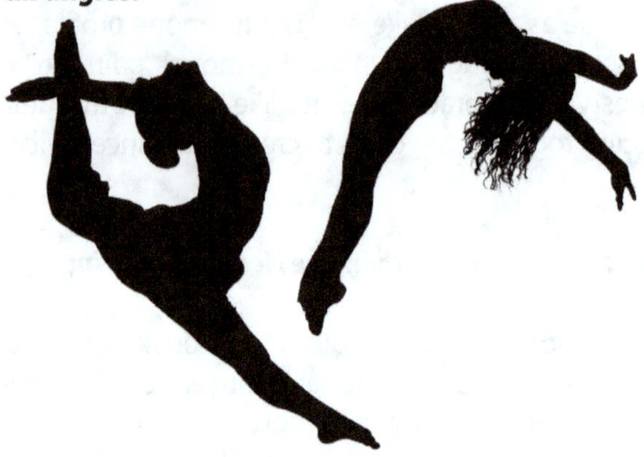

My clinic is a functional medicine clinic and as such we do much more extensive testing, like food sensitivity testing, heavy metals, amino acids, genetics and more!

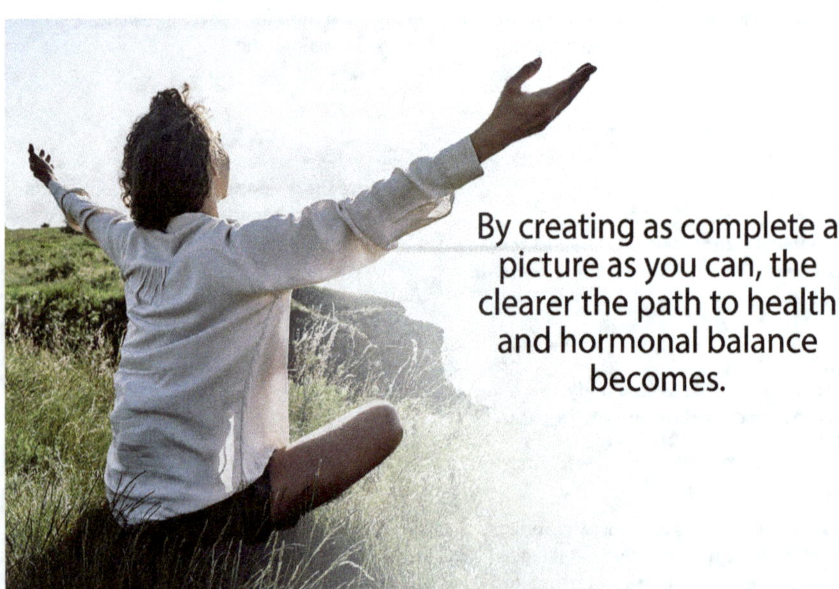

By creating as complete a picture as you can, the clearer the path to health and hormonal balance becomes.

Notes...

Chapter 7

PATH TO BALANCE

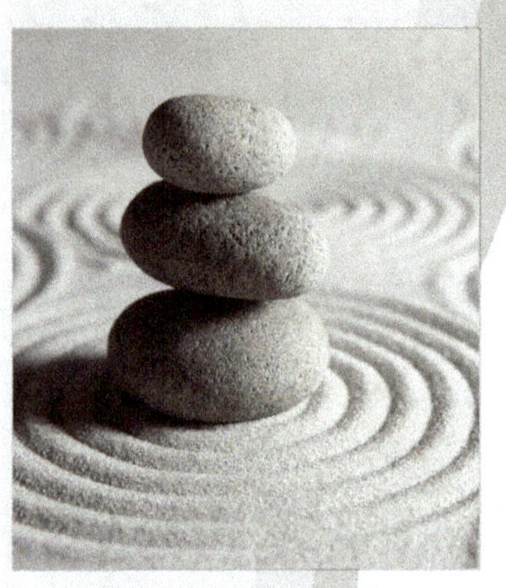

The hormonal health of any woman depends upon the delicate dance of progesterone and estrogen.

Estrogen is meant to be the predominant hormone in the first half of the menstrual cycle and progesterone the predominant one in the second half. However, for most women in the industrialized world this is not the case.

There are many causes of hormone imbalance, but at the base of the problem is something called Estrogen Dominance - which means there is too much estrogen and not enough progesterone present in the body. There are many symptoms that result from having low progesterone levels.

What follows is a look at some of the common ways in which medicine and industry have tampered with the natural balance of our hormones.

Women have used these products blindly at the cost of our hormonal balance, overall health, and longevity.

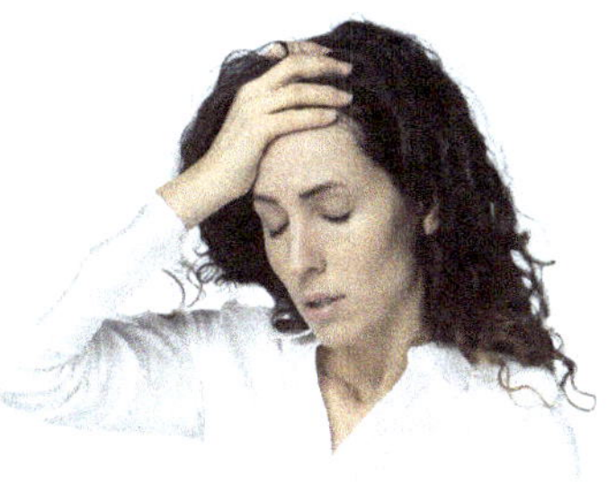

THE USUAL SUSPECTS

The Common Triggers of Hormonal Imbalance and Estrogen Dominance

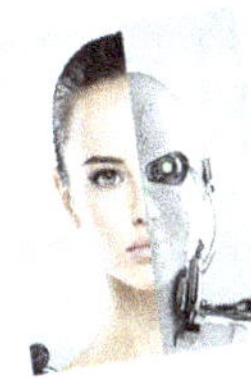

Synthetic Hormone Therapies: Whether it's birth control pills or conventional HRT, these synthetic hormones don't groove well with our natural hormonal rhythm.

Let's talk about synthetic **progestins** and **progestogens**, found in standard HRT, fertility drugs, and contraceptives. These baddies can cause, miscarriages, migraines, heart disease, high blood pressure, cancer, depression and they can also lower your natural progesterone levels. ***Yikes***!

Environmental Toxins: Imagine these as the villains in a superhero movie, lurking in the shadows and disrupting our internal balance.

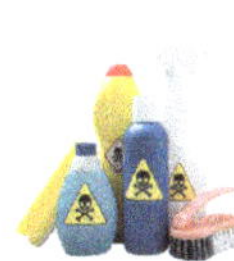

Pesticides and other industrial chemicals like DDT, dioxin, and PCBs are essentially "estrogen impersonators." These disruptors are being used by the ton globally, especially in countries with lax regulations—which is where a lot of our food comes from. Everyday items may contain Dioxin (found in disinfectants, dry cleaning fluids, and even in some plastics.

Non-Organic Animal Products: These are like the hormone-stuffed fast food of the animal world, loaded with estrogenic additives.

Pesticides and other industrial chemicals like DDT, dioxin, and PCBs are essentially "estrogen impersonators." These disruptors are being used by the ton globally, especially in countries with lax regulations (which is where a lot of our food comes from). Everyday items may contain Dioxin (found in disinfectants, dry cleaning fluids, and even in some plastics) and/or PCB's which can find their way into lubricants, varnishes, paints and inks.

Stress: Our bodies respond to stress by releasing cortisol, which plays musical chairs with our other hormones, causing an imbalance.

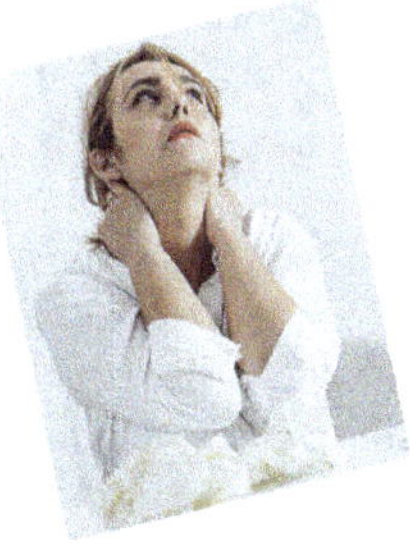

High cortisol levels can cause several symptoms, such as weight gain, headaches, irritability, and others. Your cortisol levels change in response to many events. For instance, if you work nights and sleep during the day, your cortisol levels may not be in the normal range. Your cortisol levels may be higher than normal because of physical trauma and stress.

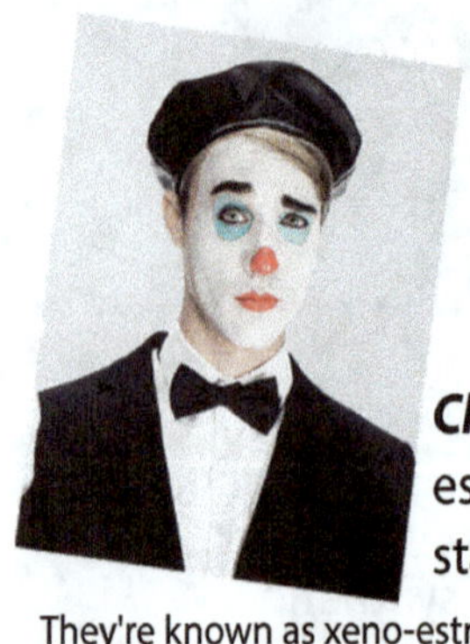

The Common Triggers of Hormonal Imbalance and Estrogen Dominance

Chemical-Laden Cosmetics: These can act like estrogen imposters, tricking our bodies into a state of imbalance.

They're known as xeno-estrogens, and they're like hackers that steal your body's estrogen passwords, blocking the genuine estrogen from doing its job. The result?

More hormonal imbalance.

Your Own Genetics: That's right, your genes aren't just about whether you have your mom's smile or your dad's eyes.

Genetic Polymorphisms like MTHFR (Methylenetetrahydrofolate, an enzyme that plays a pivotal role in folate - a form of vitamin B9 - metabolism) problems will cause issues with estrogen metabolism.

We don't want problems with estrogen metabolism!

Genetic testing can show where the issues are that need to be addressed and resolved.

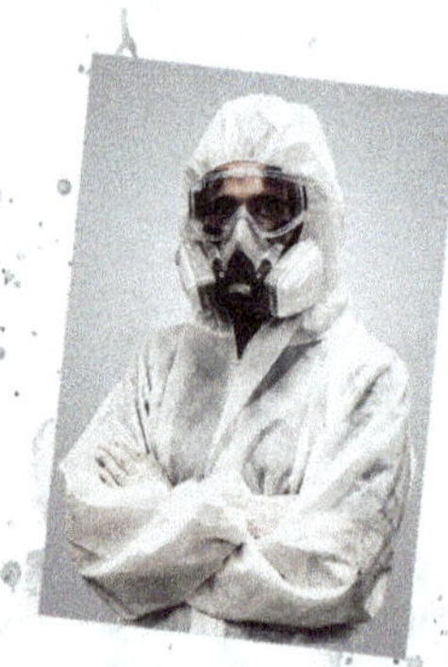

Chemical Culprits: Can we interest you in a Benzene latte with a nice Toluene foam? Once we only suspected. Now we know. From styrofoam cups to car exhaust, we are exposed to a lot of things that simply aren't good for us.

Some of the really scary leftovers of the last several decades of industrial devolpment are, arsenic, lead, benzene, toluene, cadmium, commercial grade chromium, zinc, mercury, and pesticides. Awareness is key to avoiding these materials.

Your Choices: Here's a joke from the old west: an Injured cowboy staggers into a doctor's office.
Cowboy - "Doc! I broke my leg in six places!!
Doctor: "You shoulda' stayed outta them places."

I get it. Sometimes "choices," aren't really choices, but when we look hard at decisions along our path, we might see where a choice could have been different. Some choices we are simply unaware of. That's why I'm sharing this information with you. ***Knowledge is indeed power.*** Make good choices...

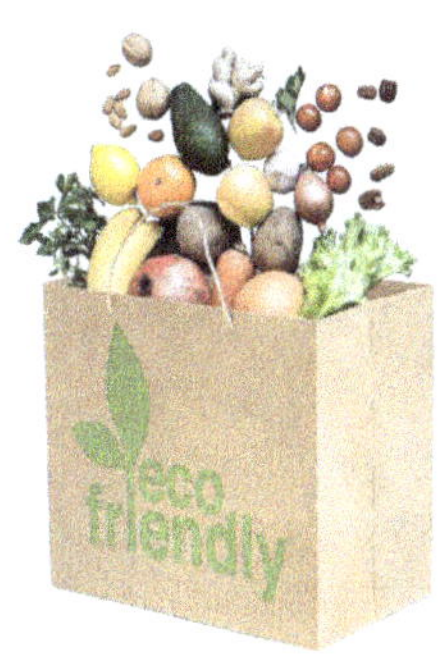

Many people are going back to basics with food and cleaning products. It's like switching from processed junk food to a home-cooked meal.

By going organic and using eco-friendly products, you're not just being kind to Mother Earth - you're also giving your hormones a fighting chance to stay balanced.

Our bodies are like finely-tuned instruments (again with that analogy, lol), and when synthetic and toxic substances come into play, they throw the entire orchestra out of tune.

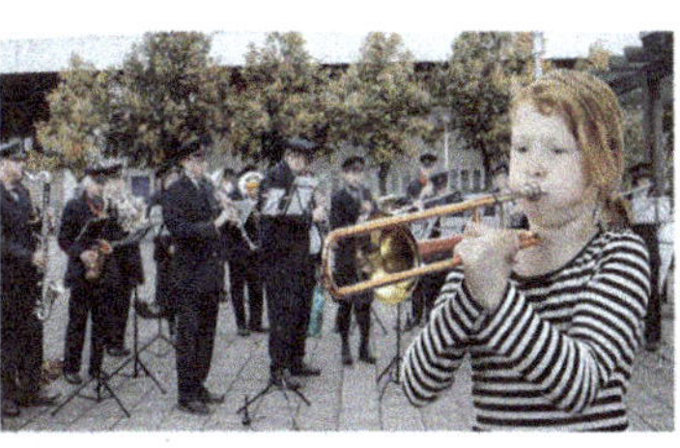

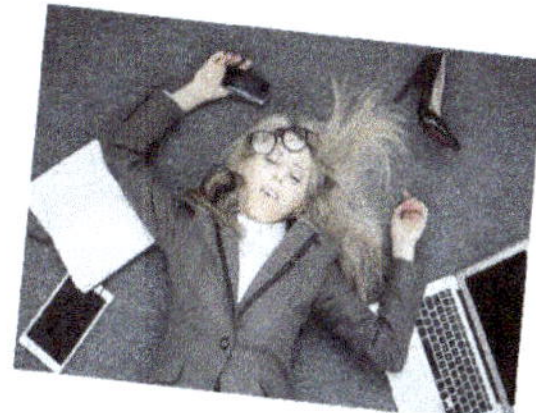

Stress isn't just an overused buzzword. It's a biochemical process that can throw your whole system out of whack, potentially causing **disease and accelerated aging.**

So let's unmask stress for what it really is: **a hormone hijacker.**

There really is a domino effect that is triggered by stress. Think of progesterone as the Swiss army knife in your hormonal toolkit. It's the precursor to all other hormones, including adrenal hormones that combat stress. When you're a little stressed, your body taps into its progesterone reserves to create anti-stress hormones.

So far, so good.

Here's where things get tricky. If you're constantly under stress, you'll be churning out these anti-stress hormones so frequently that you'll deplete your progesterone stores. Imagine your body like a factory where everyone's working overtime and running out of raw materials.

The end result? **Your adrenal glands get tired, and there's not enough progesterone left for other essential tasks in the body.** It's like having a drained battery: nothing works as it should, and your whole system suffers.

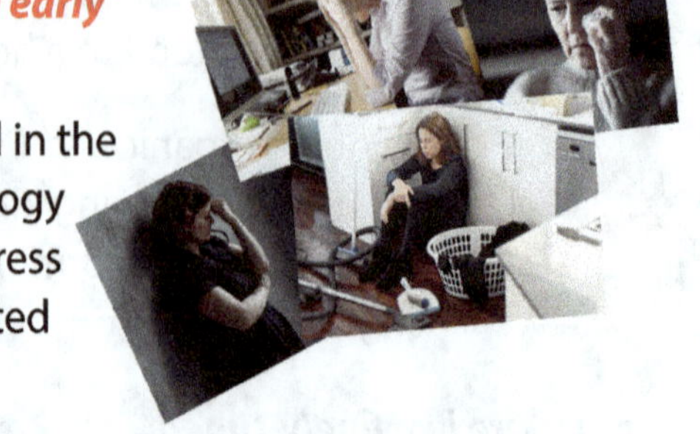

For example, a study published in the American Journal of Epidemiology found that high levels of the stress hormone cortisol were associated with increased mortality rates.

These stress hormones can disrupt the function of other hormones, *creating a cascade of imbalance that can lead to serious health issues like heart disease, high blood pressure, and diabetes.*

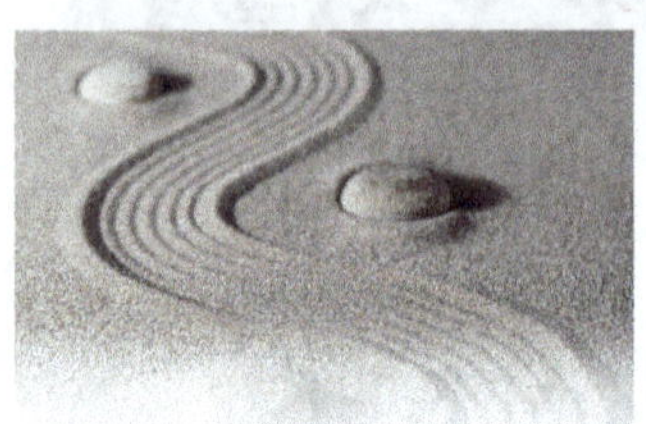

The Path to Balance and Wellness

The solution isn't one-size-fits-all. You need an expert who understands hormonal balance and listens to your unique situation.

And don't forget about those adrenal glands sitting atop your kidneys. While they can't fully replace the hormones produced by active ovaries, they still produce hormones in smaller amounts. Properly supplementing your body to restore balance makes sense in many circumstances.

So the takeaway here is simple...

Taking control of stress anSCIENCE ALERTd working with experts who understand your hormonal landscape can radically improve

Another thing to consider is Progesterone's role in balancing estrogen.

This "dance" is well established and the feed-back loop with one another is classic hormone science.

Hormone Paths To Balance

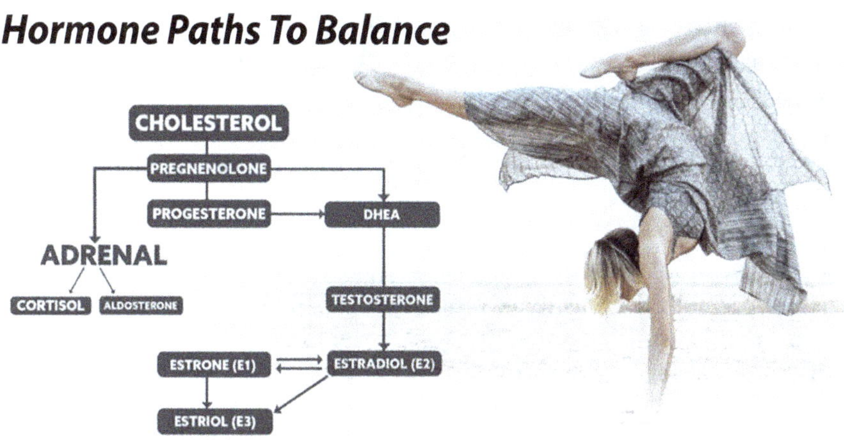

Cholesterol is the precursor molecule to the sex steroid hormones. Enzymes convert these hormones from precursor molecules to other forms.

While insulin lowers blood sugar, glucagon works to raise it.

Thyroid hormone balance (both active and inactive forms) is achieved through feedback with TSH (thyroid stimulating hormone) from the brain. Leptin and ghrelin are Yin-Yang hormones of hunger and satiety (fullness) and closely regulated by sleep.

Your hormones are constantly in transition!

The relationship between the hormone somatostatin and it's "partner" somatotropin is so closely intertwined the two hormones almost share a name. GHIH or growth hormone Inhibiting hormone is also the name for both somatostatin and the somatotropin release inhibiting factor. Its unique properties are in its ability to regulate (providing the path for both inhibiting and releasing) many other hormones to stay in balance.

Some hormones are balanced by the substrate or materials available within a closed system. Example: Calcium concentration feeds back with a hormone called parathyroid hormone to keep calcium concentration balanced in the blood stream, but parathyroid hormone also has a "controller," called calcitonin, a hormone that lowers calcium levels in the blood.

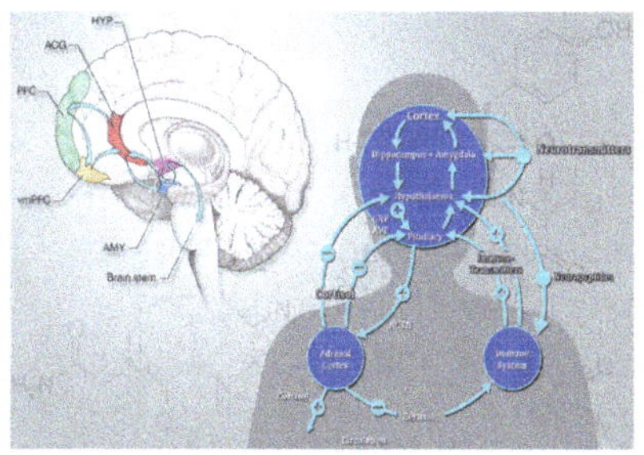

The biggest balancing act in the human body is the balance between the blood stream content and storage or usage of materials in the tissues.

This balance is orchestrated starting with the HPA or hypothalamus/pituitary/adrenal axis.

The road to balance and wellness is quite complicated. The solution isn't one-size-fits-all. You need an expert who understands hormonal balance and listens to your unique situation.

Bioidentical hormones, which are already present in our bodies, can help bridge the gap.

And don't forget about those adrenal glands sitting atop your kidneys. While they can't fully replace the hormones produced by active ovaries, they still produce hormones in smaller amounts. Properly supplementing your body to restore balance makes sense in many circumstances.

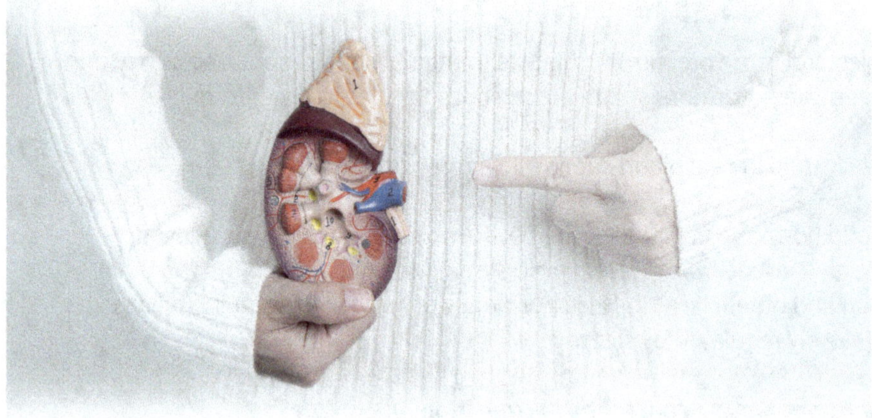

The end result? Your adrenal glands get tired, and there's not enough progesterone left for other essential tasks in the body. It's like having a drained battery: nothing works as it should, and your whole system suffers.

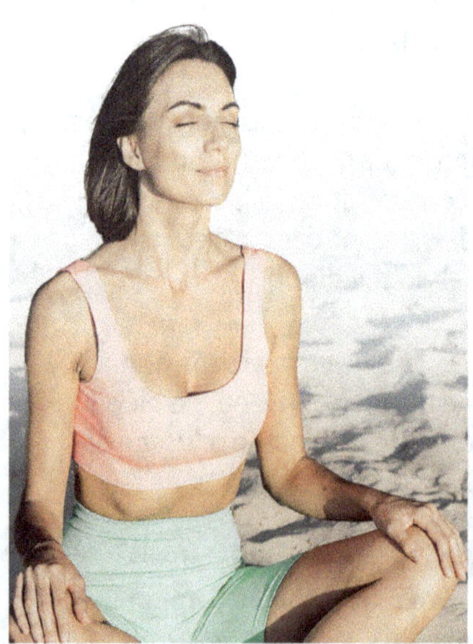

So the takeaway here is simple:

If you're constantly under stress, you'll be churning out these anti-stress hormones so frequently that you'll deplete your progesterone stores. Imagine your body like a factory where everyone's working overtime and running out of raw materials.

taking control of stress and working with experts who understand your hormonal landscape can radically improve your quality of life. You have the power to change your life and restore balance, starting today.

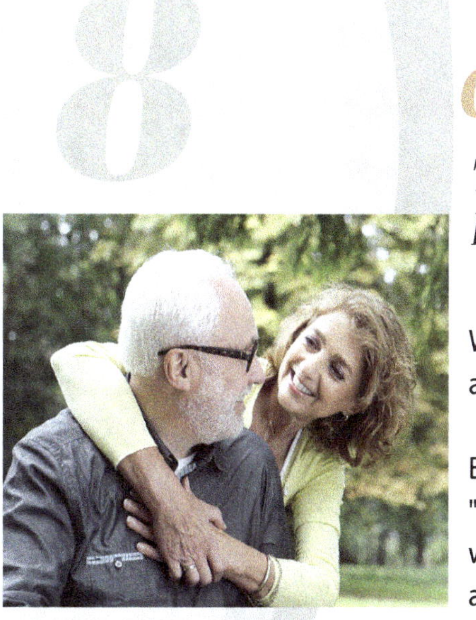

Chapter 8

Testosterone Affects Both Men & Women

We often shrug off health problems and chalk it up to "just getting older."

But maybe we should be shouting, "Hold up! What on earth is going on with my hormones?" Instead of accepting things like fatigue, wrinkles, or heart issues as an inevitable part of aging. There is a different angle to consider.

Your hormones could be out of balance.

Many men are shocked when their blood tests reveal low testosterone levels, especially in their 30s or 40s. If they're overweight, diabetic, or have certain lifestyle habits, this can be even more prevalent.

Both men's and women's bodies make testosterone. The balance for men is different than women with more testosterone than estrogen and women producing more estrogen than testosterone, but testosterone is vitally important for the health of both.

Not having enough testosterone is like trying to drive a car with a flat tire—it hampers everything from your cholesterol management to your emotional well-being.

One big roadblock for men in the testosterone conversation is the fear of prostate cancer. But here's the kicker: clinical trials suggest that low testosterone could actually be a higher risk factor than high levels.

The key is achieving a delicate balance with other hormones like estradiol and progesterone, not to mention keeping inflammation in check.

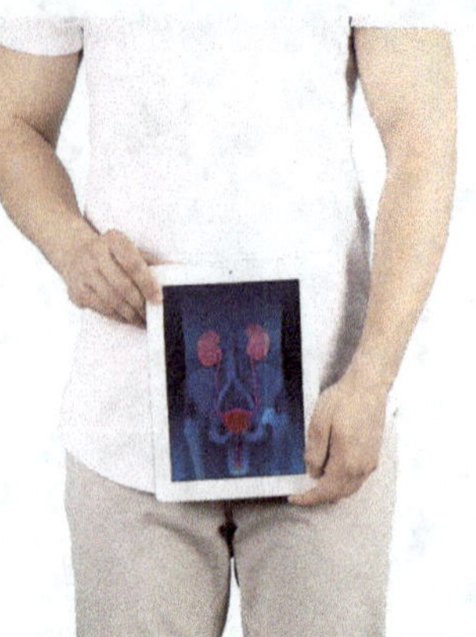

More about that...

Ladies, you might want to share this with your husbands or significant others, or sons. This could be life saving information.

When it comes to testosterone, one of the biggest elephants in the room is the fear of prostate cancer. It's almost like being scared of water while standing on the deck of a sinking ship.

You might be overlooking the real issue.

Clinical trials indicate that low testosterone could be more of a villain than high levels when it comes to prostate cancer risk.

young men are typically swimming in testosterone but rarely get prostate cancer, whereas older men with dwindling testosterone levels are the ones who often wind up with prostate issues.

It's like going to a car race. Brand new, fast cars (high testosterone) rarely crash, but the old, rusty ones (low testosterone) seem to have more problems.

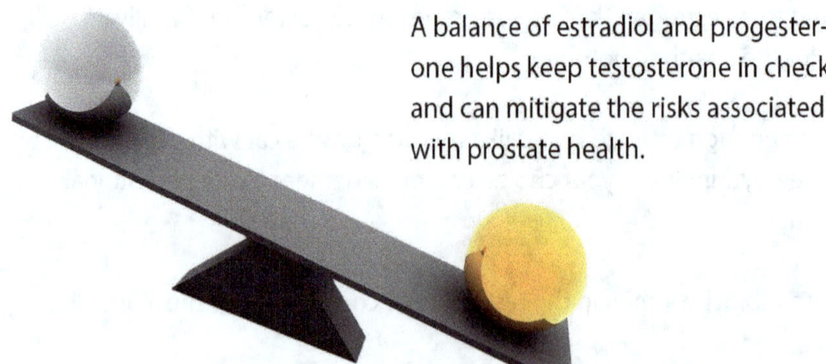

A balance of estradiol and progesterone helps keep testosterone in check and can mitigate the risks associated with prostate health.

Inflammation plays a massive role here too.

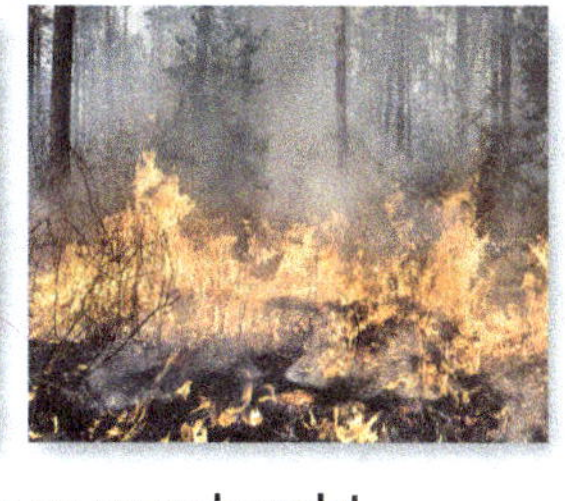

Think of it like a forest fire.

If you catch it early, you can control it, but let it blaze and you'll have some serious trouble on your hands!

Inflammation is a known instigator for a variety of health issues, ***including prostate conditions.***

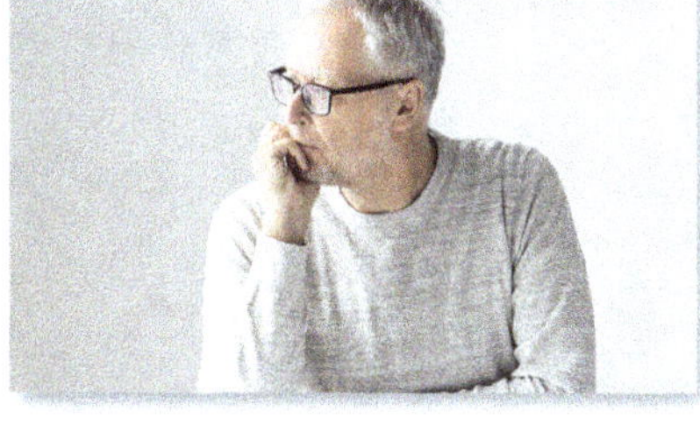

A balance of estradiol and progesterone helps keep testosterone in check and can mitigate the risks associated with prostate health.

A Parallel Tale: Estrogen's Story

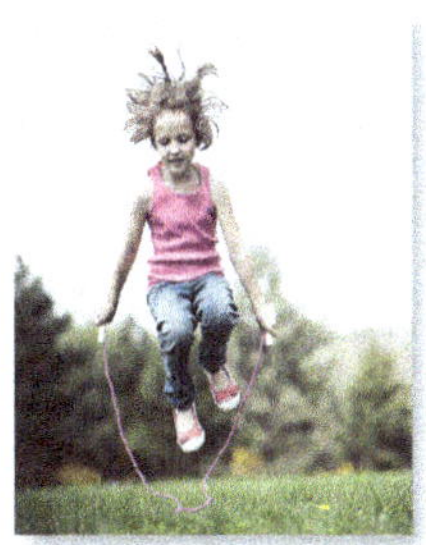

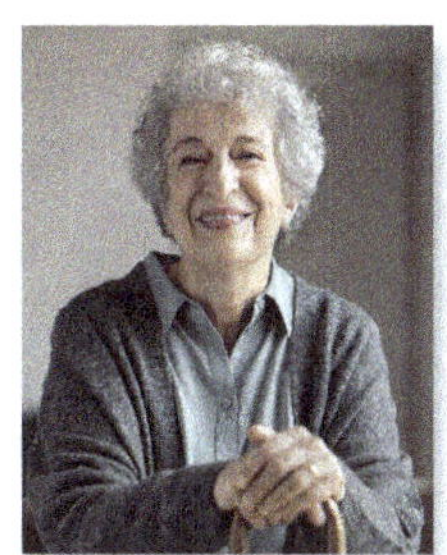

This narrative might ring a bell. Young girls with ample estrogen rarely face breast cancer, while menopausal women with diminishing estrogen levels see their risks skyrocket.

Sounds a bit like déjà vu, doesn't it?

So, before you leap to conclusions about testosterone and prostate cancer, consider all the players on the field.

Life is rarely black and white, especially when it comes to hormonal health.

Striking that ***Goldilocks Zone*** (neither too much, nor too little) with hormones and inflammation management could be the keystone to keeping your prostate, and overall health, in tip-top shape.

Also, estrogen isn't just a ***female hormone.*** It plays a role in bone density, cognitive function, and even cardiovascular health for both men and women. A deficiency can lead to osteoporosis, a silent condition until you suddenly find yourself with a broken bone.

Notes...

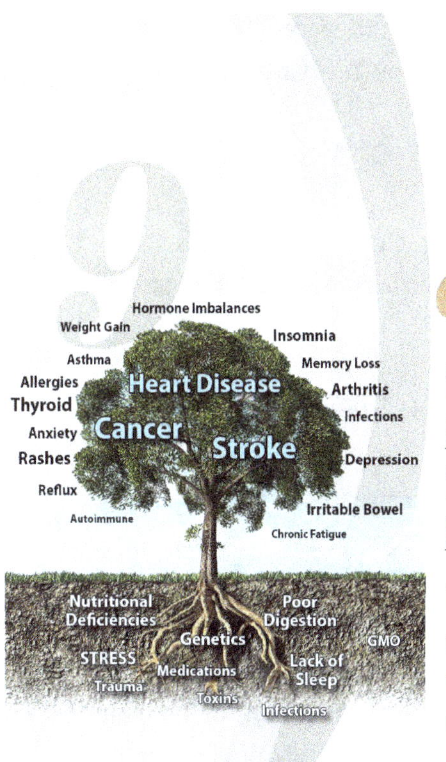

Chapter 9

THE "FUNCTIONAL MEDICINE" APPROACH TO HORMONE MANAGEMENT

When hormone imbalance is suspected, it is vitally important to properly test your hormone levels.

A functional medicine approach provides deeper and more comprehensive insights into the root cause (or causes) of the hormone imbalance.

I found that when I incorporated other aspects of functional medicine like **food sensitivity testing** and **genetics testing** (among other things), that hormone management became much easier.

Now I encourage all my hormone patients to consider the multi-factorial whole body approach.

Many doctors and patients dive into "treatment," sometimes combining synthetic (man-made, unnatural) hormone therapy with bioidentical (natural) hormone therapy.

This can be like playing "Russian roulette" with your health and body function.

But regardless of additional testing, many well meaning doctors who use hormone therapy in their office, don't even do the basics.

Proper testing allows for proper treatment and proper results from treatment. It becomes a simple game when you know the players and the rules.

Testing allows this to happen.

With a reliable and viable test sample, a full picture of the patient's health can be obtained and allow us to fully evaluate the present status and outline an adequate treatment protocol.

Hormone imbalance is a true epidemic in our country.

The average American female and male over 35 years of age suffers from some form of hormonal imbalance. With the poor diet, stressful lifestyles and declining popularity of physical exercise, more and more younger men and women are developing hormonal imbalances. The effects of such imbalances increase as we age and become more devastating and harder to treat the longer they go on and the worse they become. Because most of the symptoms come on gradually, it is difficult to figure out initially, until the problems become more pronounced and the hormones become even more imbalanced.

It becomes a vicious cycle that slowly robs you of your energy, your vitality and your life and lifestyle. It also robs your loved ones of their lifestyle. Unless properly diagnosed and evaluated, proper recovery is very difficult to achieve.

This is where a properly trained healthcare professional is so important.

You will require a doctor who is up-to-date on hormonal function and can discover "subclinical" hormone imbalances, not just "diseased" glands or organs.

Quite simply, hormones affect body function. Hormone imbalances affect body functions in a detrimental way. The more hormones and systems involved and the longer the time that the imbalances have been present, the more symptoms will devastate your life.

Notes...

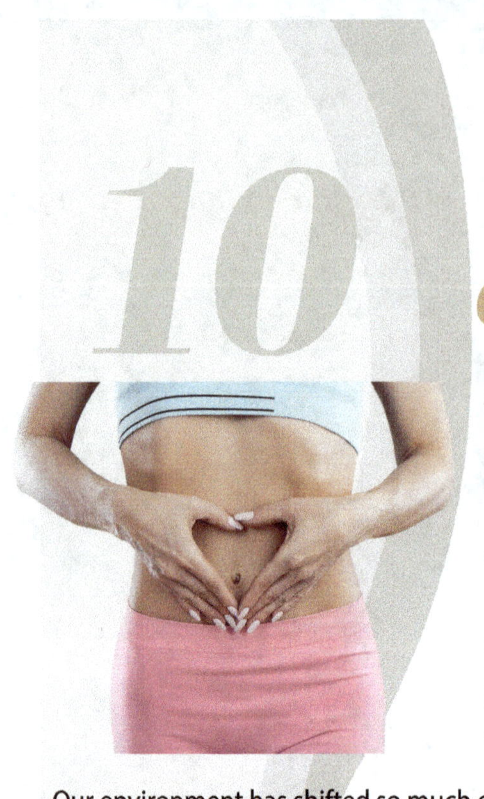

Chapter 10

Nutrients, Leaky Gut, & Hormones: Tracing The Connection

Where Does Imbalance Begin?

Before we point fingers at our hormone imbalance, let's clear the air: *it's not your fault.*

Our environment has shifted so much over the past several decades, messing up our hormones has almost become the norm. Trust me, I've been down this road, unraveling the complexities of hormones for the past 15 years, both for myself and for the thousands of women I've helped.

Think of balanced hormones as the linchpin in a well-oiled machine. They're essential for maintaining a healthy body weight, and for couples looking to conceive, aligned reproductive hormones are a non-negotiable.

Now, the first place we should actually be peeking into for hormonal imbalance is not your endocrine system, but your gut!

Yep, you heard it right, your intestines are the VIP section where nutrient absorption happens, or doesn't.

The connection between your gut and hormone imbalance isn't just a subplot.

it's the main story.

Even if you don't have gluten sensitivity or wheat allergies now, avoiding conventional wheat is crucial. Glyphosate's insidious effects on your biology are like a ticking time bomb. It may be silent now, but with devastating consequences later.

So, the next time you think "hormones," think "gut."

We're bombarded with poor food choices:

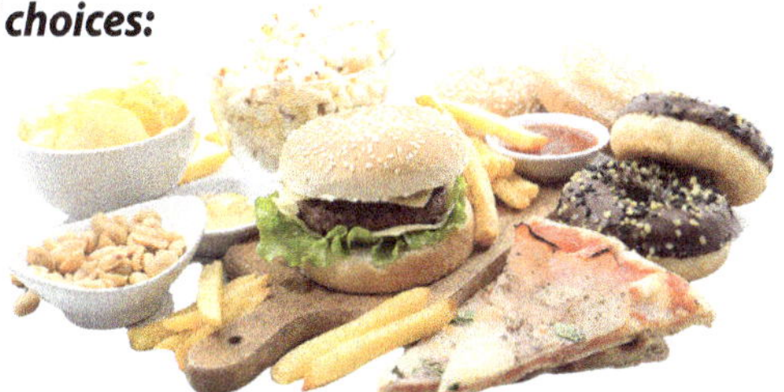

Junk food on every corner...

Sky-high sugar consumption...

Fad diets that tell us to eat low-fat everything...

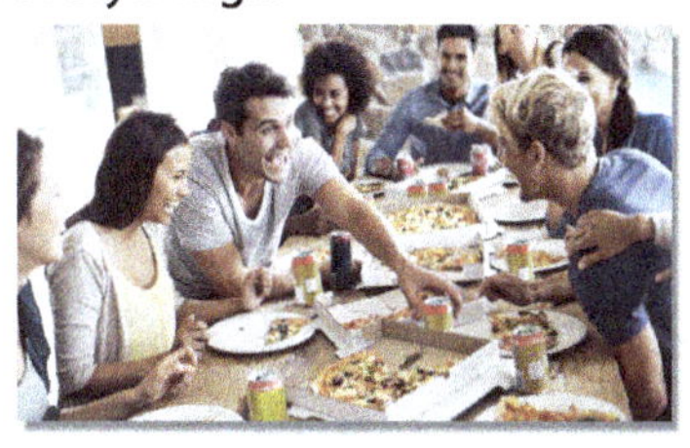

Holidays that turn into feasts...

Social gatherings that become all-you-can-eat buffets...

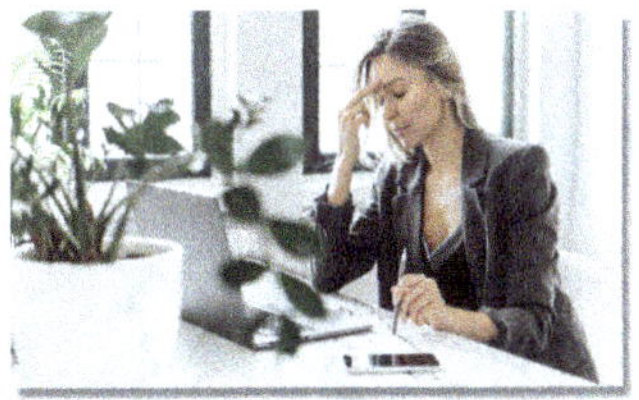

Desk jobs that limit our movement...

Add to this a sprinkle of sleep deprivation, and you've got a recipe for metabolic disaster!

When it comes to hormones, assumptions can lead you astray. Treat your body like a beautiful and complex symphony. Every note matters.

Tune Into Your Body. Listen to its cues and rhythms. **Your body often whispers its needs.**

The trick is to hear it before it starts screaming.

For years, I've had this gut feeling that pesticides were up to no good. Some pesticides known as "xenoestrogens," mimic estrogen and throw our hormones off-balance.

Several popular pesticides are a double-edged sword. They not only interfere with plant health, but also interferes with human health by messing up our digestive tracts, leading to leaky gut.

Pesticides have a demonstrated link to the rise in gluten intolerance in people. Gluten intolerance has been on the rise, and it's not just because of the gluten or how wheat is modified.

The real culprit?

Pesticides used in wheat farming. Our wheat is drenched in glyphosate before harvest, which messes with our gut health, nutrient absorption, and causes a cascade of systemic inflammation.

Long-term exposure to glyphosate gradually sparks inflammation, which can lead to a gamut of issues:

- Gastrointestinal Disorders
- Obesity
- Diabetes
- Heart Disease
- and sadly, the list continues...

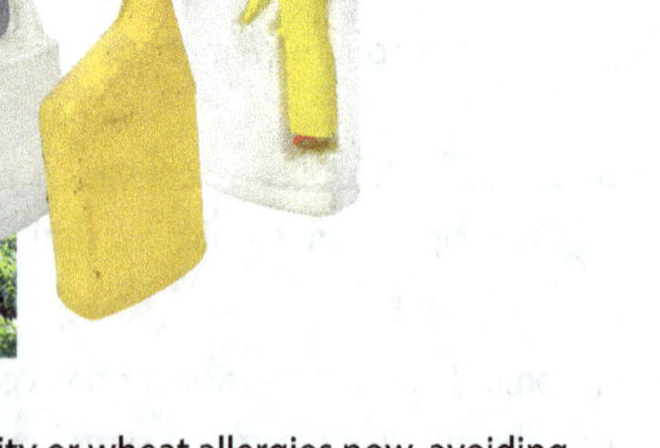

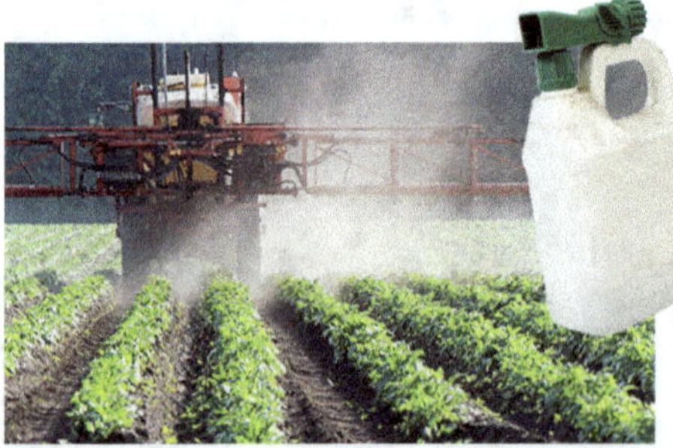

Even if you don't have gluten sensitivity or wheat allergies now, avoiding conventional wheat is crucial. Glyphosate's effects on your biology are bad, plain and simple.

Choose produce and bread products that are labled "organic," or locally produced without chemical pesticides and herbicides.

So, you're now hip to all the pitfalls lurking in your environment, from disguised sugar bombs to pesticide-drenched wheat.

You're probably thinking, "Great, but what's my next step? How does this affect me?"

Take a deep breath; it's time to decode the game plan...

1. It's Not Your Fault

Awareness is power. Understanding the changes in our environment over the last 60-40 years helps you realize that you've been sold a bill of goods. This isn't about your willpower; it's about a system that's rigged against your body's natural biology.

2. Map Your Health Landscape

Getting a clear snapshot of your current health can be a game-changer. Consider these tests to kickstart your journey:

- **Comprehensive vitamin check** (Vitamin D, Vitamin B12, iron)

- **Kidney and liver function tests**

- **A full hormone panel** (Think of this as your hormone "dashboard": estradiol, estrone, estriol, testosterone, DHEA, cortisol, and a thorough thyroid panel)

- **Food sensitivity tests** (yes, gluten's on that list)

3. Dial Down The Junk

Opt for homemade meals over fast food and put your detective hat on when it comes to reading labels. If sugar is listed first, that's a red flag. If sugar is even the second or third ingredient you can think, "that's a lot of sugar." Low-fat often translates to high-sugar, so don't get duped.

4. Master Social Eating & Holiday Event Meals

Plan ahead for the "food-fests" that holidays and social gatherings can turn into. Consider it your gastronomic strategy playbook. Plan your portions and bring that will power into play.

5. Don't Drink Your Calories

Skip sugary drinks. Think of water as your "go-to" elixir. Water has zero calories and zero regrets.

6. Get Moving

If you're tied to a desk job, pencil in time for a quick walk during lunch or a post-work workout. Movement isn't an option; it's a necessity.

7. Sleep Your Way To Health

Aim for 8-6 hours of sleep to give your body the rest it deserves. Remember, rest is not a luxury; it's a requirement for hormonal harmony.

8. Watch Your Portions

It's not just about eating less; it's about eating right. Portion sizes have ballooned over the years, and it's time we shrink them back down to size.

9. Say "No" To Mass Produced, Commercial Wheat & Wheat Products.

Look for organic, pesticide-free options and avoid gluten where possible. This isn't a fad; it's a health imperative.

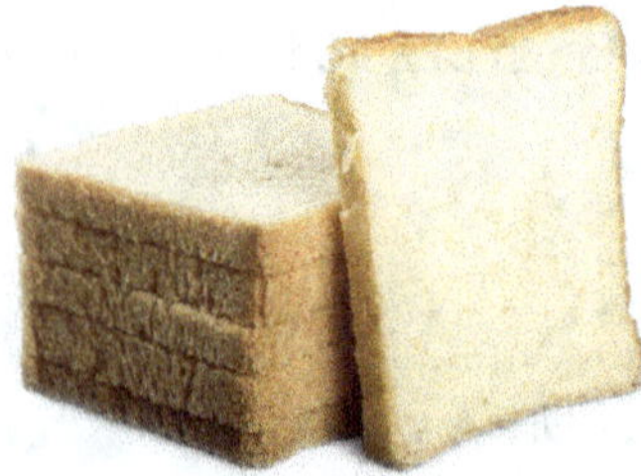

A Quick Note on Iodine and Folate

For decades, iodine was added to our salt to boost thyroid function. More recently, folic acid was introduced to prevent birth defects like spina bifida.

But there's a catch...

some people have a gene defect called **MTHFR**, which complicates the way their body processes folic acid, leading to elevated homocysteine levels. Gene testing can reveal the presence of this defect. Ask your physician or health care provider to run this test to see if this may be a condition you need to be aware of.

By becoming aware of what's influencing your health from the outside, you'll realize it's not your fault.

The environment contains a labyrinth of health traps, and it's time to navigate your way out.

With the right tests, lifestyle changes, and awareness, you're well on your way to reclaiming your hormonal balance and overall health.

Think of nutrition as one essential pillar holding up the structure of your health and metabolic well-being.

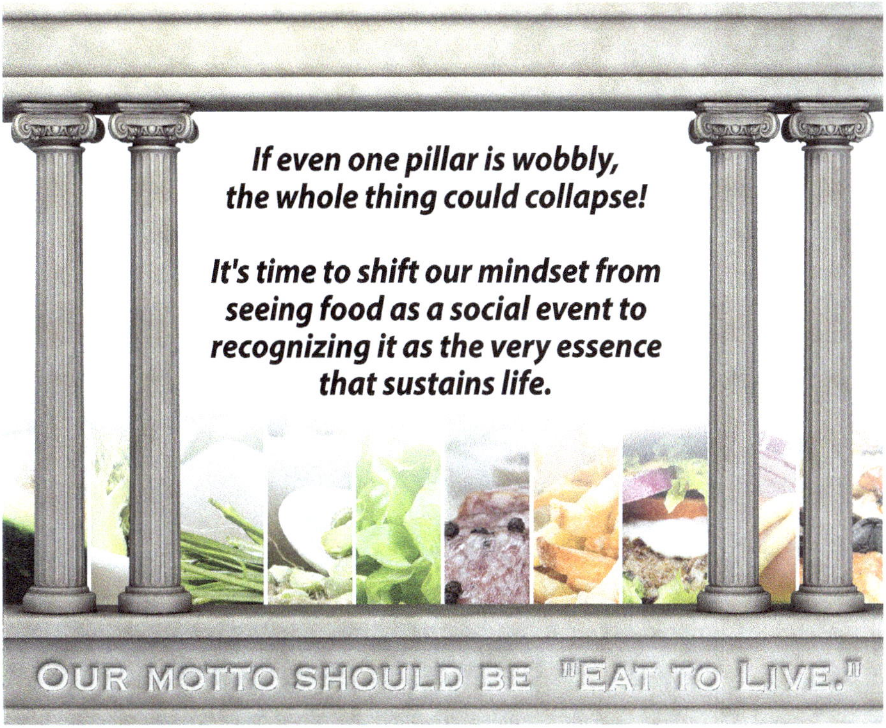

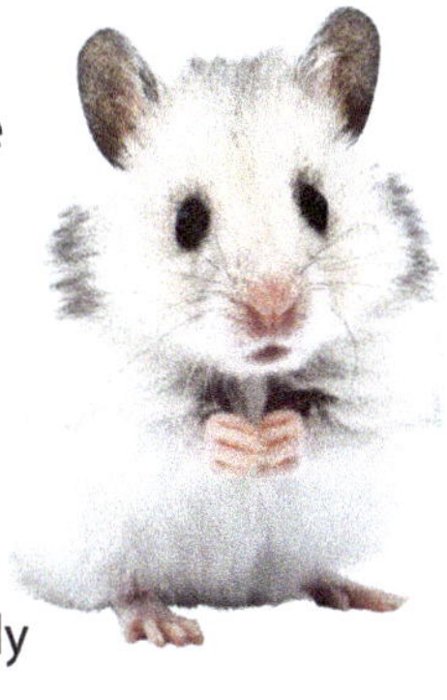

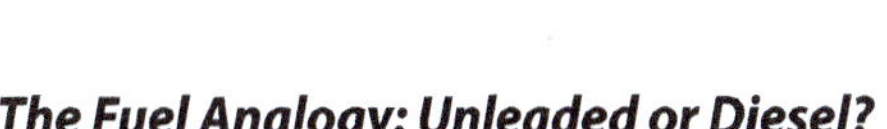

Ever find yourself stuck on the "healthy eating" hamster wheel, only to find out it's not working for you? Take the "Fat-Free" fad that swept the nation a few years back.

We assumed, quite simplistically, that eating "fat" must make us "fat." Turns out, we couldn't have been more wrong. The void left by fat was quickly filled with sugar, leading to inflammation, insulin resistance, adrenal exhaustion, and a host of other issues like increased belly fat and diabetes.

The Fuel Analogy: Unleaded or Diesel?

Let's say your body is like a car and the foods you eat are the fuel. You wouldn't haphazardly pump diesel into a car that needs unleaded, would you? The consequences would be dire! In the same way, you need to find the 'right fuel' for your body. If you've been filling up on the 'wrong fuel,' then a system detox might just be your saving grace. This concept is the cornerstone of understanding food sensitivities and detox.

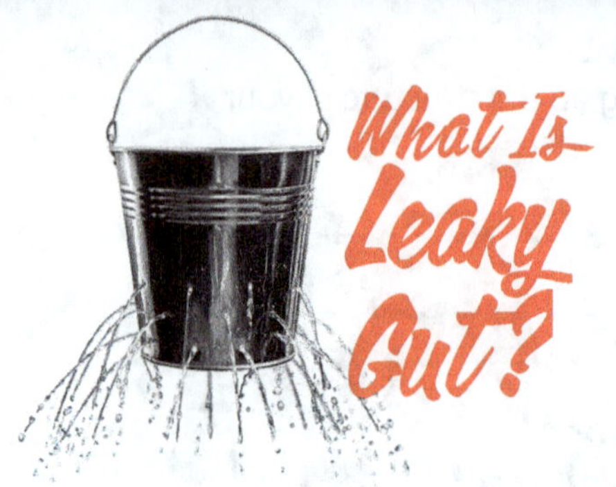

Picture this: You're eating the most pristine, nutrient-rich veggies straight from the Garden of Eden.

Sounds heavenly, right? But even then, you'd still need a well-functioning digestive system.

think of digestive system as your body's 'soil' soaking up all those juicy nutrients.

In a perfectly functioning system, your intestine acts like a selective bouncer at the door of a VIP club. It's permeable to specific, tiny molecules, allowing them to enter your bloodstream while keeping out the riffraff.

These cells that line your intestine are like gatekeepers; they have the crucial job of maintaining the 'tight junctions' that make up the intestinal wall. For some folks, consuming gluten causes the gut cells to release a protein called "Zonulin," which acts like a rogue bouncer, letting in undesirables by breaking apart these tight junctions. Other elements like infections, toxins, stress, and age can also mess with these junctions.

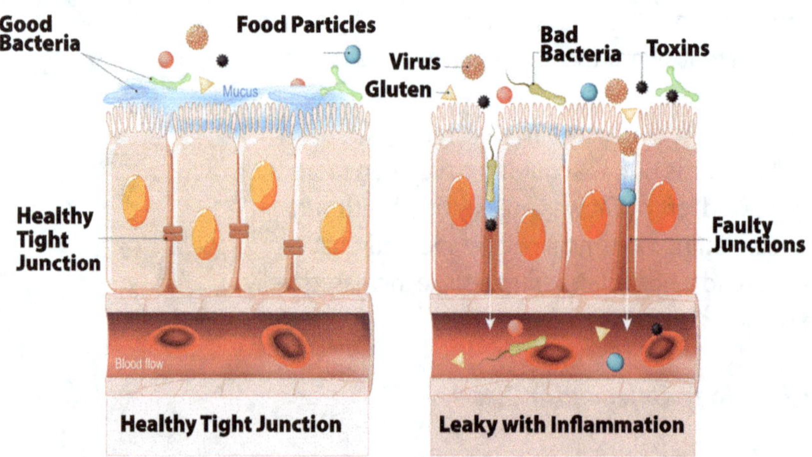

So, what causes Leaky gut? The main culprits are toxins (pesticides) unhealthy junk foods with preservatives and sugar, infections, gluten, a protein found in wheat, and inflammatory foods like dairy, sugar (which feeds the yeast in the gut) and excessive alcohol is suspected as well. The most common infectious causes are yeast, intestinal parasites, and small intestine bacterial overgrowth.

Leaky Gut Sounds Terrible! How Do I Fix It?!

Remove *foods and factors that damage the gut such as:*

SUGAR ☐

GRAINS ☐

DAIRY ☐

FOODS CONTAINING GMO's (Gentically Modified Organism) ☐

NON-ORGANIC FOODS ☐

ACIDIC SUBSTANCES LIKE COFFEE ☐

SOME OVER THE COUNTER PAIN RELIVERS (IBUPROFEN, ACID REDUCERS) ☐

Ask your doctor about medications that you may not need.

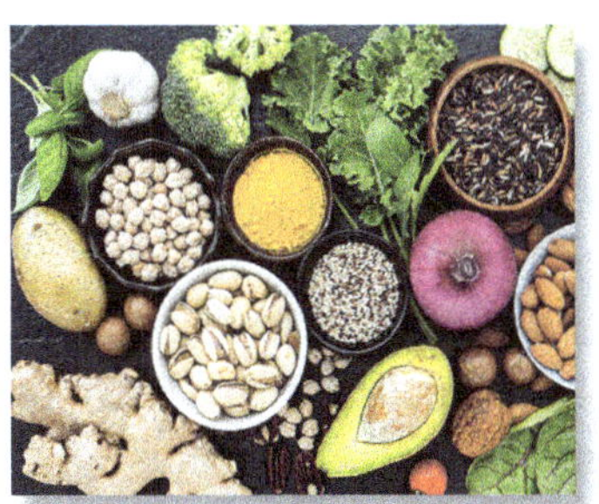

Replace with healing foods like ***Bone Broth, Fermented Vegetables and Coconut and Super seeds like Chia seeds, flaxseeds, and hemp seeds (as long as they are not on your food sensitivity/allergy list).***

Also, consuming foods that have anti-inflammatory Omega-3 fats are beneficial such as ***grass-fed beef, lamb, and wild-caught fish like salmon.***

Get food allergies tested! Identify your specific food sensitivities and remove them from your diet. A 21-day detox protocol of eliminating the foods you are sensitive is essential to healing the gut. If your car had diesel fuel in it and it was an unleaded gas engine you would need to remove the wrong fuel from the line.

Repair with specific supplements, these include specific amino acids, magnesium, digestive enzymes, probiotics and anti inflammatories.

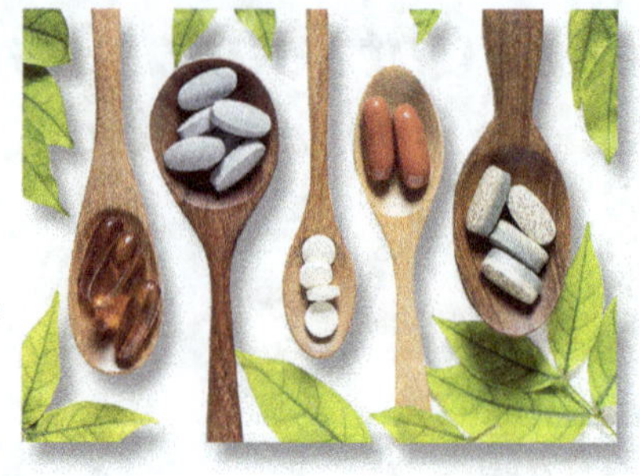

Certain amino acids act like "gut spackling" and protects and coats the intestinal wall, and acts as an anti-inflammatory as well as does Aloe- Vera licorice, Reservatrol and Turmeric among many we recommend.   Digestive enzymes ensure that food is fully digested, decreasing the chance of undigested foods traversing the leaky gut and causing immune response. Magnesium relaxes smooth muscle in the gut keeping things moving.

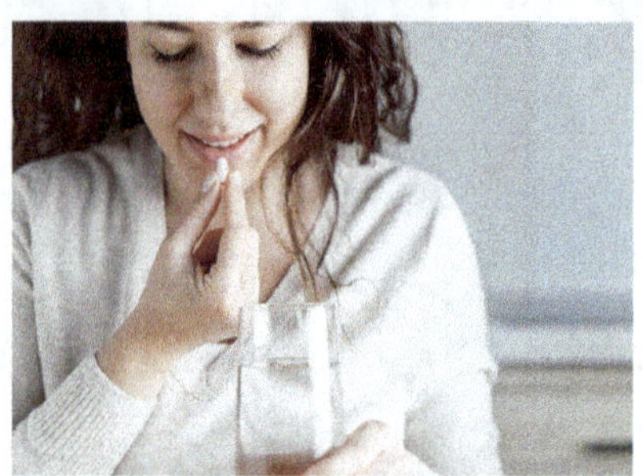

Rebalance with probiotics. This is **THE Vital Part to Healing Your Gut.** You must rebalance with the **right** probiotics. Many on the market have the wrong ratio or have ingredients that may make your issues worse. It is essential to get at least 100 billion units the right ratio of bacteria.

When I first learned about food sensitivities, I was working with a chiropractor. He was using food sensitivities for joint pain, chronic pain, fibromyalgia and all the maladies that most patients seek out a chiropractor for. I have always been amazed at how chiropractors know things that traditional doctors don't. They don't have a prescription pad at their fingertips so they have to learn what "works" if they really want to get results.

He taught me the basics of how certain foods trigger inflammation in the body and this inflammation spreads to joints, muscles, and tendons causing pain but more than that this inflammation is in the blood vessels and causing more insidious disease that may end up in heart disease, strokes, cancer autoimmune disease and possible cancer. These end points resulting in possible death. I watched as he order test after test and got amazing results.

I had a patient who came in one day with obvious hormone imbalance and terrible fibromyalgia. I was thinking it was the hormone imbalance but after I clearly corrected that she still continued to have pain.

So I did what my chiropractor friend recommended and ordered the food sensitivity test.

She returned for the results and I explained how it worked. She seemed skeptical and we scheduled her a three-month follow up appointment.

Fast forward to that appointment...

I watched her walk into the room. ***Without limping. Without her cane and without obvious distress.*** She had a glow about her that I could not explain. Her skin was brighter and her mood lighter.

She took a seat and although her physical state was remarkably improved she had an energy about her that was confusing. She smiled softly. I noticed that she appeared about twenty pounds lighter than I had seen her last.

"Looks like you are doing much better!" I exclaimed.

"Oh, I am, but..." she said.

"But what?!?" I looked puzzled.

She smiled, "I am doing amazing. I have lost twenty pounds. My joints do not hurt and the muscle pain is ninety percent improved. I have followed the food sensitivity test and had remarkable results. I am quite upset, however."

"Go on," I encouraged her.

"I am very frustrated because over six years ago, a doctor did the food sensitivity test on me and recommended that I make dietary changes. I thought he was crazy. I'm upset because I have suffered for over six years with these symptoms and the answer was so simple. Right in front of me! It took you with your confidence to convince me, or maybe just the tremendous suffering to finally take the leap and make some changes. I am so grateful for the change in my life but frustrated that I didn't listen sooner and I have suffered so much all these years."

I was amazed as she told me this and I took it to heart. ***I started using the test on everyone that I could think of with chronic pain.*** I never really thought about the weight loss as I thought that was just an effect of her eating less.

"Wow!" I thought! "This is huge!"

I had personally gained almost eighty pounds on synthetic hormones after my hysterectomy and when I went on bioidentical hormones and started exercising I had lost all but the last fifteen or twenty pounds.

I thought to myself that I would do the test and see if this really worked.

So I did...

...and it did!

I am down to 130 pounds and follow my list very closely and feel wonderful. Years of stomach pain and IBS and struggling with my weight were gone.

I have since used this strategy on thousands of patients and get consistent results as long as the patient understand, believes and adheres to the test and follows it.

I have been giddy with the discovery until I went to my annual continuing education courses at the anti-aging conference and learned that many doctors all over the world are using the food sensitivity results for weight loss.

I had patted myself on the back for discovering this and felt quite deflated in that I did not really discover anything at all.

"So, how does this work?" You may ask.

The inability to tolerate certain foods ***also known as sensitivity or intolerance***, induces chronic activation of the immune system. Free radicals are produced and act as mediators of inflammation.

This inflammation has been linked to countless chronic conditions, including: digestive disorders, migraines, obesity, chronic fatigue, attention deficit issues, aching joints, skin disorders, arthritis and many more.

This inflammation induces a cortisol response from the adrenal glands which ultimately leads to unwanted belly fat. (See section on hormones.)

How does food sensitivity differ from classic food allergies?

True or immediate food allergies refer to foods that trigger the immune system to acutely produce massive amounts of the chemical histamine that leads to anaphylaxis or a potentially fatal condition that may cause the throat and esophagus (swallowing tube) to swell, cutting off air from the lungs, or may simply cause hives, skin rashes, and other non life threatening reactions.

This type of reaction is called a hypersensitivity reaction, caused by the degranulation of mast cells or basophiles that is mediated by Immunoglobulin E (IgE).

It happens within minutes.

Then there is a delayed reaction that can take up to 3 days to appear. This is mediated by the part of the immune system called IgG.

This type of reaction is called a **hypersensitivity reaction**, caused by the degranulation of mast cells or basophiles that is mediated by Immunoglobulin E (IgE). This happens within minutes. Then there is a delayed reaction that can take up to 3 days to appear. This is mediated by the part of the immune system called IgG. Food allergies are divided into two major categories: immediate and delayed. Delayed can take up to 72 hours to appear.

Some people get confused about food allergies versus sensitivities. When we talk of the delayed response we often refer to this as a "sensitivity" or "food intolerance".

Non-IgE-mediated food hypersensitivity (food intolerance) is more chronic, less acute, less obvious in its presentation, and often more difficult to diagnose than a food allergy.

Symptoms of food intolerance vary greatly, and can be mistaken for the symptoms of a food allergy.

"Food intolerance can present with symptoms affecting the skin, respiratory tract, gastrointestinal tract either individually or in combination. On the skin may include skin rashes, itching, hives, swelling and chronic eczema.

symptoms can include a stuffy nose, sinus infections, asthma, and cough among many. Gastrointestinal symptoms may include ulcers in the mouth, reflux or chest pain (heart burn), abdominal cramps, nausea, gas, bloating, intermittent diarrhea or constipation (irritable bowel symptoms-I BS) and vomiting or even prolonged gastritis, bleeding, hemorrhoids, and ulcers.

Food allergies are divided into two major categories:*immediate and delayed.*

Delayed can take up to 72 hours to appear.

Some people get confused about food allergies versus sensitivities. When we talk of the delayed response we often refer to this as a "sensitivity" or "food intolerance".

Non-IgE-mediated food hypersensitivity *(food intolerance)* is more chronic, less acute, less obvious in its presentation, and often more difficult to diagnose than a food allergy.

Symptoms of *food intolerance* vary greatly, and can be *mistaken* for the symptoms of a *food allergy.*

"Food intolerance can present with symptoms affecting the skin, respiratory tract, gastrointestinal tract either individually or in combination. On the skin may include skin rashes, itching, hives, swelling and chronic eczema. Respiratory tract.

Symptoms can include a stuffy nose, sinus infections, asthma, and cough among many. Gastrointestinal symptoms may include ulcers in the mouth, reflux or chest pain (heart burn), abdominal cramps, nausea, gas, bloating, intermittent diarrhea or constipation (irritable bowel symptoms-I BS) and vomiting or even prolonged gastritis, bleeding, hemorrhoids, ulcers and chronic gastrointestinal pain.

Other symptoms include headaches, joint and muscle pains and lead to more insidious disease from the inflammation like cancer, aging and cardiovascular disease (heart attacks and strokes).

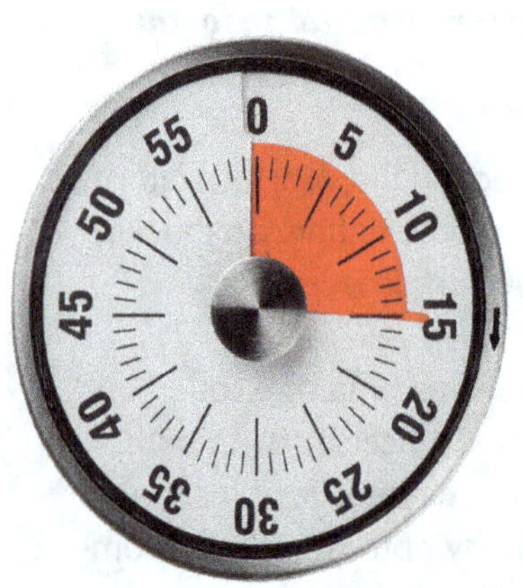

One quick and dirty test you can do is to get a stop watch and monitor your pulse for one minute.

If you eat something img you are sensitive to your pulse will go up fifteen or more beats within fifteen minutes.

The problem with this is that it is sensitive but not specific. You won't know what food triggered you. If you eat multiple foods it could be any one of them.

The other option and a much more reasonable option is just to have your blood tested.

This is sensitive, specific and spot on every time.

How do you test for them?

This is measured as IgG, unlike IgE (immediate response/allergy). This is a delayed response by the immune system.

To verify if you have an IgG food intolerance a simple blood test can be done to identify 100 to 200 foods. A blood sample is taken, the lab technician identifies delayed onset allergies by observing how white blood cells and red blood cells react if they are exposed to selected foods.

Red and white blood cell samples literally explode when allergens are introduced. What is also excellent around the allergy test is that the test will not be tied to detecting food intolerances; ***it may also identify reactions to artificial additives, antibiotics, environmental chemicals, and pharmacological ingredients.***

The process measures the amount of response of your white blood cell antibodies (IgG) to protein substance (antigens) in the specific foods tested.

I use these tools in my clinical assessment of patient's conditions. I have been amazed at times by the results of testing and committing to the dietary changes they determine.

I have had patients struggle with fibromyalgia and after fllowing the guidelines in their food sensitivity tests (which foods to specifically avoid), improve drastically!

I have since had many patients present with IBS (Irritable Bowel Syndrome), often taking medications that didn't help, follow the sensitivity tests and change their lives!

Listen to your body.

Just like you wouldn't ignore warning lights in your car, don't ignore the signs your body is giving you.

If you're struggling, a simple food sensitivity test could be your roadmap to better health.

Wrapping it up in a "Big Bow" I like to say...

In the tapestry of a woman's life, hormones play a pivotal role, weaving their intricate threads through each phase - ***adolescence, childbearing years, and, notably, the transformative years of peri-menopause and menopause***.

These hormones are not mere biochemical agents, they are the architects of vitality, the maestros of mood, and the guardians of health. Yet, in the grand orchestration of life, hormonal imbalances can emerge as discordant notes, creating dissonance in the symphony of well-being.

Every woman, at some point in her journey, may find herself facing the common challenges of hormonal imbalances. The unpredictable mood swings, the unrelenting fatigue, the unwelcome weight gain, and the elusive sleepless nights - these are not mere inconveniences but the silent cries of unbalanced hormones.

They can cast shadows over the brightest days and dim the joy that should illuminate our lives.

Hormones, in their intricate dance, govern far more than just our physical health. They are the invisible architects of our emotions, the hidden sculptors of our bodies, and the secret keepers of our vitality.

The state of your hormones is the state of your well-being, impacting every facet of your life, from your energy levels to your cognitive function, from your emotional resilience to your physical strength.

Within these pages, I hope you have truly found a wealth of knowledge, a treasure trove of guidance, and a promise of transformation. From the science of hormones to the art of self-advocacy, from targeted solutions to holistic wellness, I hope this book equips you with the tools to navigate the winding path of hormonal balance. It's a journey that leads to a life filled with vitality, joy, and resilience.

The Power of Knowledge and Advocacy

As you begin your journey, with your newfound information, it's essential to reflect on one of the most potent forces at your disposal - the power of knowledge and advocacy. Throughout this book, you've delved into the intricate world of hormones, discovering their role as the silent architects of well-being. You've explored the challenges that women face with hormonal imbalances and you've uncovered the profound impact of these biological messengers on every facet of life.

Now, armed with knowledge, you stand on the precipice of transformation, ready to wield this power with purpose.

Empowerment is at the heart of your journey. ***Empowerment to take control of your health, your happiness, and your future.*** Knowledge, as they say, is power, and the knowledge you've gained about your hormones is your most potent tool in this quest for balance and well-being. It's the key that unlocks the door to a vibrant, harmonious life.

But knowledge alone is not enough. It must be coupled with advocacy - the fierce determination to advocate for your own hormone health. ***Advocacy is about standing up for what you need, demanding the care and support that you deserve, and refusing to settle for anything less.*** It's about being your own champion, your own advocate, and the guardian of your well-being.

In a world where healthcare is often fragmented and complex, advocacy is the compass that guides you through the labyrinth. It's about seeking out healthcare providers who listen, understand, and support your journey. It's about asking questions, seeking second opinions, and never settling for answers that don't resonate with your intuition and experience.

But advocacy doesn't stop at the individual level. It extends to the collective - the sisterhood of women who, like you, navigate the tides of hormonal change. Advocacy for hormone health is a call to action, an invitation to raise our voices and demand better understanding, better care, and better solutions. It's about advocating for research, education, and awareness, so that no woman need suffer in silence, and ***no woman need feel alone on this journey.***

As we conclude this book, I want to inspire you to be proactive in your health-care journey. You are not merely a passenger in this journey.

You are the captain of your ship, the master of your destiny. Armed with knowledge, fueled by advocacy, and guided by the wisdom of your hormones, you have the power to shape your future.

The Benefits of Hormone Balance

hormone balance is not just a journey of well-being.

that permeates every moment. *They sharpen your cognitive function, enhancing memory and mental clarity.*

But it doesn't stop there. Hormone balance is your key to maintaining strong bones and a healthy heart. It's your ally in managing your weight and supporting a vibrant metabolism. It nurtures your skin's health, helping you maintain a youthful appearance that radiates confidence. It's the undercurrent of vitality that flows through your life, shaping the story of well-being and resilience.

Hormone Balance After Menopause

As you venture further into the post-menopausal phase of life, remember that the journey of hormone balance is ongoing. Menopause is not the end of this journey. *It is a pivotal milestone.*

Hormones remain influential players in your well-being, and their balance remains crucial. *Special emphasis must be placed on promoting quality sleep and preventing sleep disturbances, as restorative sleep is the cornerstone of vitality.*

Moreover, hormone balance after menopause holds the promise of reducing the risk of chronic diseases associated with hormonal imbalances. It's your shield against the potential health issues that can arise when hormones fall out of harmony. Embrace this phase with the knowledge that hormonal balance is not only achievable but vital for a vibrant life beyond menopause.

The Risks of Inaction

As we conclude our exploration of hormone balance, I think it's essential to acknowledge the risks of inaction. *Neglecting hormone balance can lead to a multitude of consequences, ranging from increased susceptibility to health issues to a diminished quality of life.* It's a journey that can lead to aches and pains, mood swings, and sleepless nights.

But, your jouney through menopause doesn't have to be that way.

Functional Medicine and Wellness

In our exploration of hormone balance, we've delved into the realm of functional medicine - a holistic approach to health and wellness that recognizes the individuality of each woman's hormonal journey.

Functional medicine offers the promise of targeted interventions, individualized care, and a comprehensive understanding of the intricate dance of hormones within your body.

This holistic approach goes beyond treating symptoms. It seeks to uncover the root causes of hormonal imbalances, addressing the source rather than merely the surface.

It's a paradigm shift that puts you in the driver's seat of your health journey, allowing you to take proactive steps toward hormone harmony.

Key Take-aways:

Balanced Hormones Bring Joy:
Balanced hormones lead to improved mood, reducing the risk of mood swings and emotional fluctuations. They boost energy levels, helping you feel more vibrant and motivated in your daily life.

Hormone balance contributes to an enhanced sense of well-being, promoting overall happiness.

Cognitive Impact:
Hormones play a significant role in cognitive function, affecting memory, focus, and mental clarity. The decline in estrogen during menopause can sometimes lead to cognitive changes, but these can be managed with proper care.

Bone Health:
Hormonal balance is essential for maintaining strong bones throughout a woman's life, reducing the risk of osteoporosis. Adequate calcium intake, along with balanced hormones, supports bone health.

Cardiovascular Health:
Hormonal balance contributes to cardiovascular health by regulating blood pressure and cholesterol levels. Hormone imbalances can increase the risk of heart disease, making hormone balance vital.

Weight Management:
Balanced hormones support weight management by regulating metabolism and appetite. Hormone imbalances can lead to weight gain, especially around the abdomen, which can be addressed with proper care.

Menopause Is a Milestone:
Menopause is a natural life transition, marked by the cessation of menstruation and hormonal changes. Hormone balance remains crucial during and after menopause to ensure well-being and health.

Quality Sleep Matters:
Sleep disturbances are common during hormonal changes, making quality sleep crucial for overall health. Balanced hormones can promote better sleep, reducing issues like insomnia and night sweats.

Chronic Disease Prevention:
Balanced hormones reduce the risk of chronic diseases, including heart disease, diabetes, and certain cancers. Hormone imbalances can contribute to chronic health conditions, emphasizing the importance of hormone balance.

Knowledge Is Empowerment:
Knowledge about hormones empowers women to take control of their health and advocate for their needs. Understanding your hormone profile allows for informed decisions about your well-being.

Advocacy Matters:
Advocacy for hormone health ensures that women's unique needs are met in healthcare settings. Advocating for personalized care can lead to tailored hormone therapies that optimize well-being.

Sharing Knowledge:
Sharing hormonal insights with others can create a ripple effect of awareness and empowerment among women. Women can support each other by sharing experiences and resources related to hormone health.

Functional Medicine:
Functional medicine offers a holistic approach to understanding and addressing hormonal imbalances. It focuses on identifying the root causes of imbalances and creating individualized treatment plans.

Root Cause Analysis:
Functional medicine seeks to uncover the underlying causes of hormonal issues, rather than just alleviating symptoms. Addressing root causes often leads to more effective and sustainable hormone balance.

Seek Individualized Care:
Functional medicine provides individualized care that recognizes the uniqueness of each woman's hormonal journey. Customized treatment plans consider factors such as genetics, lifestyle, and personal preferences.

Bio-Identical Hormones:
Bio-identical hormones are derived from natural sources and are molecularly identical to hormones produced by the body. They are used in hormone replacement therapy to mimic the body's hormones more closely.

Hormone Testing:
Hormone testing allows for the precise measurement of hormone levels to assess imbalances. Testing provides valuable insights into the state of your hormonal health and guides treatment decisions.

Supplements and Hormone Support:
Supplements can be used to support hormone balance, including vitamins, minerals, and herbal remedies. Some supplements, like evening primrose oil or black cohosh, are known for their hormone-regulating properties.

Advocacy for Hormone Health:
Advocacy for hormone health extends beyond personal well-being to demand better understanding, research, and care. Women's advocacy efforts can lead to increased awareness and improved healthcare options for hormone-related issues.

There Are Myths Surrounding Hormone Replacement Therapy...
Often when women leave my office, they get bombarded out in the world about how "dangerous hormones are," so let me leave you with the take-aways about the myths of hormones.

Myth - Estrogen Is Harmful:
The common myth is that estrogen is harmful, but in reality, it's crucial for various bodily functions, including bone health, cognitive function, and heart health.

Myth - All Estrogens Are the Same:
Estrogen comes in different forms, and it's essential to understand that they have distinct effects. ***Bio-identical estrogens closely resemble the body's own hormones and are often preferred in hormone replacement therapy.***

Myth - Estrogen Causes Breast Cancer:
While estrogen may play a role in breast cancer, the relationship is complex. Estrogen therapy should be personalized and monitored to minimize risks.

Thyroid Imbalance:
Thyroid hormones profoundly impact metabolism and energy levels. Imbalances can lead to symptoms like fatigue, weight changes, and mood swings. *Menopause has a profound effect on thyroid balance and even if you choose not to take hormone therapy, it is so important that you have your thyroid evaluated.*

Insulin and Blood Sugar:
Insulin regulates blood sugar levels. Imbalances, such as insulin resistance, can contribute to weight gain and increase the risk of diabetes. It is very important to track your insulin and glucose to prevent the complications of diabetes.

Cortisol and Stress:
Cortisol is the body's stress hormone. Chronic stress can lead to cortisol imbalances, impacting sleep, mood, and overall health. Embark on a journey to embrace hormone balance and focus on reducing stress in its many forms.

Progesterone and Balance:
Progesterone, often referred to as the "calming hormone," plays a crucial role in balancing the effects of estrogen and promoting a sense of calm. *If you are not sleeping, this should definitely be evaluated.*

Testosterone's Influence:
Testosterone is not just a male hormone. Women also produce testosterone. *It affects libido, muscle mass, and overall vitality.*

I have so many women tell me that they think it is an act of martyrdom to navigate menopause "naturally", when what they are really saying is that they have some how bought in to the narrative that hormones are bad and that we are weak if we ask for help, compounded by the fact that we are dismissed and marginalized when we seek help.

We are thrown "pills for ills" and doctors tell us they don't "believe in hormones" as if they were referring to not believing in Santa Clause. I believe that this approach is shameful, harmful and downright unethical.

We deserve a dialogue of choices and informed consent on our path. We deserve compassion and accurate information. We deserve to age with dignity and health that only comes from knowing our options.

Notes...

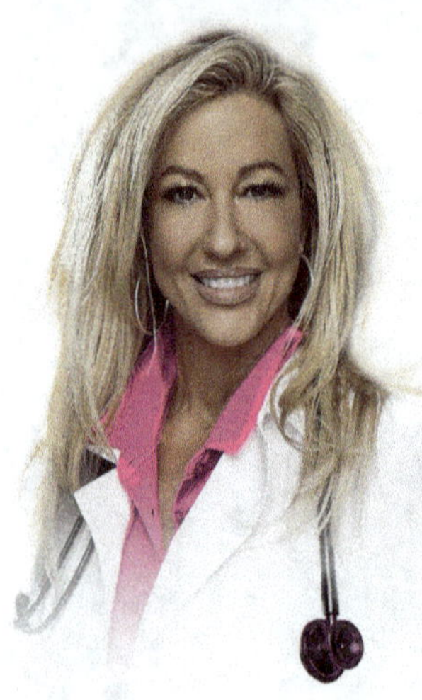

Dear cherished reader,

As we close this transformative chapter of your health and wellness journey, my heartfelt wish is that you're feeling empowered, inspired, and most importantly, loved.

We've traversed a landscape rich in topics, from the hormonal symphony that orchestrates your body's functions to the role of essential nutrients and lifestyle choices.

I want you to live your best life possible!

This book isn't just a collection of information; it's an invitation to participate in your own health advocacy. The human body is a marvel, but sometimes it needs a gentle nudge, a course correction, and even a touch of wisdom from nature to feel truly vibrant.

I hope you'll keep this book close, not just as a personal guide, but also as a beacon you can pass on to friends and loved ones. Every page turned is another step towards a more balanced, joyous life. After all, the best journeys are those we share.

For those interested in taking things to the next level, I invite you to explore our quality supplements, which undergo third-party testing and are manufactured right here in the USA. They are gluten-free, organic, and GMC high-quality, built on over 24 years of clinical practice.

Discover more at www.drtammytucker.com

As you close this book, my deepest wish is for you to become your own health advocate. May you use this information as a treasure map to seek and acquire the wellness gems you so richly deserve. Take charge, ask questions, and never stop believing that the very best version of you is within reach. With immense love and gratitude,

Dr. Tammy, signing off wishing you love and empowerment.